# Testimonials for *Juicing, Fasting, and Detoxing for Life*

Due to a huge amount of stress over the years as a priest and fire and police chaplain, I had gained about fifty pounds, almost without realizing it. Facing hip replacement and feeling tired like an old man, I tried all kinds of diets hoping that would help. I'd lose some weight, but I kept gaining it back. Then I discovered Cherie's juicing and cleansing program. I have now lost about forty-one pounds! Sometimes I replace two meals with juice and that's all I want. It's taken away my cravings— no more desire for junk foods, high-carb foods, or desserts. No more struggling! My energy level has shot up and people are always commenting on the weight I've lost and how great my skin looks. I no longer feel twenty years older than my age, but twenty years younger! —*Father Tryphon, age 61*

When I was feeling hopeless about my hypothyroid condition and the extra twenty pounds I was carrying, my naturopathic doctor told me I had to do a detox. He said it was the only way to get my body back in balance and off of thyroid medication. So, I did a serious detox with mostly raw food and the juice diet, along with some supplements, and finally, after trying for years, I dropped twelve pounds effortlessly in just months. It made a believer out of me! I didn't realize that toxins are stored in fat and that the body holds onto fat for our protection. Get rid of the toxins; get rid of the fat. I don't think I could have lost the weight without going to mostly raw foods and juice and cleansing. I didn't know that detoxing was such a critical part of shedding stubborn fat. —*Trudy, 49*

At age thirty-nine, I was so unhealthy I thought I'd be dead before I turned fifty. I felt sick all the time, tired, and had severe pain in my abdomen and lower back. At forty-one, I was diagnosed with colon cancer, which spread to my liver, lungs, and other areas of my body. The doctors didn't give me hope of recovery. That was when I found Cherie's juicing and cleansing program. First I went on the three-week alkalizing diet. Four days into the colon cleanse, my body got rid of a mass about the size of my fist. I continued to go to the clinic for monitoring, and, surprisingly, my tumor markers repeatedly went down and down. At the same time, I started feeling better and better. My energy returned. My pain went away. And I started looking healthier. I'm now forty-seven, and my doctors finally pronounced me *cancer free*! I've never felt better in my life! Recently, I ran up a flight of stairs like a teenager. When I look in the mirror, I'm truly amazed at how much younger I look. Just the other day a lady told me I looked about thirty-seven. I know my great health, youthful appearance, and my life is due to a program of juicing, alkalizing, and cleansing.                                    —*Barbara, 47*

I've lost about twenty-five pounds since I started my juicing, raw foods diet, and cleanse program. A year before, I'd set a goal to lose twelve pounds and just couldn't do it. Then I went on the juicing and raw foods program to focus on optimum health because I was diagnosed with breast cancer. Surprisingly, the weight just fell off. I eat a lot of food—all good food, and a high percentage of it is raw. And I'm not hungry at all. I have lots of energy. But the best news is that my tumor markers have fallen to half the score I started with. And I feel better than I have in years. I look younger, my hair is thicker, and my skin is clear.                          —*Nancy, 60*

# JUICING, FASTING, AND DETOXING FOR LIFE

# JUICING, FASTING, AND DETOXING FOR LIFE

Unleash the Healing
Power of Fresh Juices and
Cleansing Diets

◆

Revised and Updated

## CHERIE CALBOM, MS, CN,

### with JOHN CALBOM, MA

GRAND CENTRAL
Life & Style

NEW YORK • BOSTON

The information and advice herein is not intended to replace the services of trained health professionals, or be a substitute for medical advice. You are advised to consult with your health care professional with regard to matters relating to your health, and in particular regarding matters that may require diagnosis or medical attention.

Grand Central Life & Style
Hachette Book Group
237 Park Avenue
New York, NY 10017

www.GrandCentralLifeandStyle.com

Printed in the United States of America

RRD-C

Revised Edition: February 2014
10 9 8 7 6 5 4 3 2

Grand Central Life & Style is an imprint of Grand Central Publishing.
The Grand Central Life & Style name and logo are trademarks of Hachette Book Group, Inc.

The Hachette Speakers Bureau provides a wide range of authors for speaking events. To find out more, go to www.HachetteSpeakersBureau.com or call (866) 376-6591.

The publisher is not responsible for websites (or their content) that are not owned by the publisher.

Library of Congress Cataloging-in-Publication Data
Calbom, Cherie.
   Juicing, fasting, and detoxing for life : unleash the healing power of fresh juices and cleansing diets / Cherie Calbom MS, CN, with John Calbom, MA. —Revised.
     pages cm
   Includes bibliographical references and index.
   ISBN 978-1-4555-2135-7 (pbk.) —ISBN 978-1-4555-2136-4 (ebook)
   1. Detoxification (Health)   2. Fruit juices.   3. Vegetable juices.   4. Fasting. I. Calbom, John.   II. Title.
   RA784.5.C35 2014
   613.2—dc23

                                                                              2013021697

# Contents

◆

# Introduction

Would you like to be healthy, happy, and energetic? Want to look younger and more vibrant? How about losing some weight? Or do you need help healing your body? If you said yes to any of these questions, rest assured. The programs in *Juicing, Fasting, and Detoxing for Life* have helped thousands of people lose weight, get rid of cellulite, look healthier, soften wrinkles and lines, gain energy, restore health, prevent disease, and feel years younger.

If you have a health issue, this can be your opportunity to discover not only what contributed to your ill health, but also what will enable you to become healthier than before and live an exciting, fulfilling life of purpose. Even if you don't have any particular ailments, you can experience more energy and greater vitality along with disease prevention by using juicing, short juice fasts, and periodic detoxes for various organs of the body.

I first wrote about juicing in 1992 in my best-selling book *Juicing for Life*. Nearly two million people have read *Juicing for Life* and my sequel, *The Juice Lady's Guide to Juicing for Health*. Exciting testimonies have poured in from people all across America and around the world whose lives changed for the better when they started juicing, cleansed their bodies, and changed their diet. The "live foods" I recommend, such as fresh vegetable juices, green smoothies, and raw foods, give life to the body. And the yummy recipes allow for delicious and varied menus. I'm convinced the juicing and cleansing programs I've developed have saved my life by helping me recover from debilitating illness and injury. And I know they'll make a big difference for you, too.

The programs in *Juicing, Fasting, and Detoxing for Life* go far beyond salads and V8 juice. In fact, juices that are canned or bottled have been pasteurized, which means that many of their life-giving nutrients, such as enzymes and vitamins, have been killed in the process. And while these processed options are better than soft drinks, they fall quite short when compared with freshly made juice. But there's another important reason to drink fresh juice. It's broken down into an easily absorbable form, which makes it superior even to eating whole vegetables when it comes to absorbing vitamins, minerals, phytonutrients, and enzymes. Plus, you'd probably never eat in one day all the vegetables you could juice. Live foods like fresh juice, green smoothies, green salads, and other raw foods, along with a diet of whole foods, offer an abundance of nutrients. That's due in part to the biophotons—the light rays of energy the plants absorb from the sun. Photons feed the mitochondria—the energy units of your cells that produce ATP, your energy fuel. These foods make your body feel alive!

The programs in *Juicing, Fasting, and Detoxing for Life* include short juice fasts and specific cleanse programs that act similar to spa treatments, but on the inside. They're somewhat like a housecleaning crew for your organs and fluids, on down to your cells. Juicing, fasting, and detoxing can help you get well if you're ill and make you even healthier if you're well—perhaps more vibrant and energetic than you ever thought possible. And that means when you lose weight using these programs, you'll look healthier—you won't look drawn or washed-out as many people do on other plans. I've seen remarkable results for people attending my juice and raw foods cleanse retreats. People have arrived sick, looking ashen, with dark circles under their eyes. In just one week, they have changed dramatically. They leave with color in their faces, dark circles gone, and glowing. Nearly everyone loses between 5 and 15 pounds. Amazing!

There are many detox programs on the market, and many focus on items to purchase. Very few programs have detailed menu plans with plenty of delicious recipes that make them easy to follow. Though a few of my cleanse programs need certain herbs or other cleanse agents to make them the most effective, many of the programs can simply be followed with recipes you prepare.

In the chapters that follow, you'll find the plans that turned my life around—from illness, debilitation, and disability to good health and a desire to help others be well. I want to share with you my own journey to health and wholeness to encourage you. If I could get well and stay healthy, there's hope and the opportunity for you to do the same.

## A Health Crisis

Though I'd never been particularly healthy as a child and adolescent, I encountered a true health crisis when I turned thirty. I developed a severe case of chronic fatigue syndrome that forced me to quit my job in Hollywood and move home to Colorado with my father and stepmother. I was simply too sick and tired to do much more than lie around most of the time. I would often sleep for twelve hours at a time and still feel tired when I got up. Severe fatigue became a way of life. There were mornings when I'd get up feeling so weak that I could barely walk down the hall. I felt as if I had a never-ending case of the flu with continual swollen glands and a low-grade fever. My body ached as if I'd just been bounced around in a washing machine. And I had a severe case of candidiasis along with parasites (determined by a stool test) and heavy-metal toxicity (determined by a hair analysis). My life seemed hopeless.

I'd not been able to find a doctor who could give me anything to improve my health or any hope of feeling better. I finally went to a health food store and browsed around. I talked with employees and bought some health books. I discovered there was something I could do.

I totally changed my diet and started juicing every day. I eliminated all animal products, including dairy, along with all junk food, sugar, and wheat products. I started with a five-day juice fast. On day five, I felt much better. In the weeks that followed, I completed several other short juice fasts of two or three days and several cleansing programs. But instead of feeling better, I started feeling a little worse. Though I didn't understand the process at the time, I was detoxing. Detoxification is the process of removing toxins, which are substances that are harmful or poisonous to the body. They create irritating or injurious effects internally, undermining our health and stressing our biochemical and organ functions. Removing them doesn't happen on a wide scale without our assistance through nutritional intervention, cleansing programs, and dietary changes.

Family members were skeptical about my self-designed health journey, but I forged on with my whole foods diet, juicing, and cleansing programs. I also saw a reflexologist (a person who massages feet and applies pressure to certain parts of the foot for healing). He suggested I try a gallbladder flush because of the pain I experienced when pressure was applied to a specific area of my foot. The gallbladder detox produced rather astounding results, and I did get a little better. But I still often felt sick and tired.

Then one day, in a totally unexpected development, I woke up feeling brand-new—with energy to spare. I wanted to go jogging. That was a first. I'd made a significant turn for the better, and though my new health seemed to appear suddenly, it had been building for quite a while. I'd been on my health program for about three months. And I thought, "Wow! That was the greatest cure on earth." I realized that freshly made vegetable juices, green smoothies, lots of raw foods, periodic cleansing, and a nutritious, whole foods diet was a lifestyle I should follow for life to produce the health I wanted. I also realized there were foods I needed to let go of, like sweets, flour products such as bread and pasta, and dairy products, so I could maintain my high level of wellness.

Armed with a juicer, a new lifestyle, and an exciting set of goals, I returned to Southern California and my friends. For nearly a year, it was ten steps forward with renewed, sparkling health and more energy and stamina than I'd ever remembered.

Then, all of a sudden, I took a giant step back.

## Another Crisis

I was house-sitting in a lovely Southern California neighborhood for vacationing family friends and working on my first book. A burglar broke into their home one night. I was shocked to wake up around three a.m. and see a strange young man in the bedroom crouched in the corner. Instead of running out the open door, he attacked me, beating me repeatedly with a pipe, yelling, "Now you are dead!" and then choking me unconscious. I felt my spirit leave, floating up and out of my body. Then all was still. I sensed I was traveling, at what seemed like the speed of light, through black space, with twinkling lights in the distance. Suddenly, however, I was back in my body, outside the house, screaming for help. I don't know how I got there.

I suffered serious injuries to my head, neck, back, and right hand, with multiple head wounds and part of my scalp torn from my head. I also incurred numerous cracked teeth that required several root canals and crowns to repair. But my right hand sustained the most severe injuries, with two knuckles crushed to mere bone fragments that had to be held together by metal pins, and six months after the attack, I still couldn't use it. The cast I wore, with bands holding up my ring finger, which was almost torn from my hand (it had remained attached by only a small portion of skin), looked like something from a science-fiction movie. I felt and looked worse than hopeless, with the top of my head shaved, red, swollen eyes, a gash on my face, a useless right hand, terrorizing fear, and barely enough energy to get dressed when I woke up.

I decided I'd be a survivor, not a victim. So I went to work on getting well again. This time, it took every ounce of my will, deep spiritual work, alternative medical help, extra vitamins and minerals, juicing, emotional release, forgiveness for the attacker, and numerous detox programs to heal physically, mentally, and emotionally.

I met a nutritionally minded physician who had healed his own slow-mending broken bones with lots of vitamins and minerals; he gave me vitamin cocktail IVs. Juicing, cleansing, nutritional supplements, a nearly perfect diet, and prayer, along with physical therapy, helped my bones and other injuries heal. But the restoration of my right hand was truly a miracle.

After about six months, what my hand surgeon said would be impossible became real—a fully restored, fully functional hand. He'd told me I'd never use my right hand again and that it wasn't even possible to put in plastic knuckles because of its poor condition. But my knuckles did indeed re-form, and the function of my hand returned. A day came when he told me I was completely healed, and though the doctor admitted he didn't believe in miracles, he did say, "You're the closest thing I've seen to one."

Equally important in the restorative process was the healing of my soul—a place where no one could determine the degree of injury. I experienced healing from the painful memories and trauma of the attack through prayer, laying on of hands, and deep emotional healing work. It seemed like endless buckets of tears had been pent up in my soul from old wounds, such as my mother's death when I was six, my grandfather's death when I was nine, a tragedy concerning my dad when I was thirteen, and the attack. All that pain needed release. Forgiveness and letting go came in stages and were an integral part of my total healing. I had to be honest about what I really felt and willing to face the pain and toxic emotions stored inside and let them go. But finally I was free. A time came when I could celebrate the Fourth of July (the anniversary of the attack) without fear.

Finally, I knew more peace and health than I ever thought possible. I experienced what it was to feel whole—complete, not damaged, broken, wounded, or impaired, but truly healed and restored to wholeness in body, soul, and spirit. And I knew there was a purpose for my life—a reason I had lived. I could help others find their way to wholeness.

## You Can Enjoy Vibrant Health

Because of my health struggles and the long journey to wholeness by a road of trial and error, I wrote this book for you—wherever you're at in your pursuit of good health and vitality. You may be healthy and just want to gain a little more energy, lose a few pounds, and bolster your immune system so you don't get colds or flu as much. You may have a health condition you want to improve. Or you may have a life-threatening illness or serious injury and you want to do your part in getting well. Whatever you want to achieve, I know that you can make significant improvements in your health by following the programs in *Juicing, Fasting, and Detoxing for Life*.

I'm sharing with you what I've learned on my path to health and wholeness, as well as what I've studied in scientific research and in earning a graduate degree in nutrition, along with what I've discovered through years of counseling people regarding nutrition and their health. I've seen hundreds of people achieve near perfect health and get rid of a host of ailments, aches and pains, and even life-threatening diseases through juicing and following the various cleanse programs in this book. There's no magic bullet in this process—it's all about giving your body what it needs to heal and stay healthy along with getting rid of what hinders the healing process— the toxins, congestion, and acid buildup. As you remove toxicity, which interferes with health and healing, and give your body an abundance of life-giving nutrients like those found in fresh juice, your body can do what it was designed to— heal and stay healthy and trim.

In the chapter on mental and emotional cleansing, my husband, John, shares the knowledge he's gained about mental and emotional detox. Through his graduate work in counseling psychology and more than thirty years of working with groups and individuals regarding the care and healing of the soul, he's gained tremendous insights on letting go of mental and emotional toxicity that blocks health and healing, and he teaches you how to restore the soul.

Keep in mind that as you embark on your journey to vibrant health, it will take trust, patience, and endurance along with action to get good results. Restoration and preservation of your health come with time and persistence. If you stick with the programs in *Juicing, Fasting, and Detoxing for Life*, you will have a healthier body and soul. Your body was intended to function well. If you have physical ailments, remember that your body was designed to heal. It's important to provide the best internal environment possible so it can do its work of healing. Remember, it's taken awhile to get to where you are, so it may take awhile to correct your health issues. Take heart! You'll reach your goal if you don't give up. And while you're on your journey to vibrant health, be aware that any problems you face can be part of the weave of your new life of wholeness, vitality, and purpose—the purpose for which you were created.

You can begin your journey today by taking the first step—whatever that may be for you. Maybe you need to purchase a juicer or just simply go shopping for fresh, organic produce, or make a decision that you're going to do things that are really good for your body from this day forward. Whatever you need to do to get started, take that step today.

## Juicing and Cleansing Programs That Get Results

Make fresh vegetable juicing a part of your routine—it can be life changing! Juice fast occasionally. Some people like to vegetable-juice fast one day a week; others choose to fast one or two days each month or once a quarter. Make sure you cleanse the organs of your body once or twice a year, or optimally, once a quarter—cleanse your colon, liver and gallbladder, and kidneys. If it makes sense to change the oil and filters in your car regularly, doesn't it make sense to cleanse your body's filter systems? Be sure to stick with the cleanse programs even if you feel a little worse initially. As you clear toxins from your body, you may not feel so great before you feel better. But when you've completed the detox programs, you'll feel like a new person.

The same goes for cleansing the soul. As you clear mental and emotional toxicity from your mind and emotions, you may have to face unpleasant memories and old wounds, emotional pain may surface, and buried memories may be revealed. But the results are worth the effort. Nothing can compare with the deep peace, joy, and healthier body that come from a balanced soul.

You'll find the chapters in *Juicing, Fasting, and Detoxing for Life* to be informative and easy to follow. In chapter one you'll discover the secrets of vibrant health. Chapter two introduces you to the world of juicing and gives you guidelines for using fresh juice for vitality, energy, healing, and detoxing your body. It also gives you lots of tips for purchasing a juicer that's easy to use and clean; a blender won't work for juicing, but you'll use one for green smoothies and cold soups. Chapter three tells you all about the benefits of fasting and how to begin with a one- to three-day vegetable-juice fast that will greatly accelerate any weight-loss or health program you choose. Chapter four gives you an overview of detoxification and explains why it's so important to your health. Various detoxification protocols follow in chapters five through seven, with juices, green smoothies, cold soups, raw foods, and supplements for the colon cleanse, liver and gallbladder cleanse, and kidney cleanse, along with various specialized cleanses for *Candida albicans*, parasites, and heavy metals. Chapter eight guides you through detoxing your mind and emotions. Chapter nine follows with an A-to-Z guide that gives you a list of the foods that are highest in nutrients from vitamin A to zinc. And the last chapter gives you dozens of delicious juice and green smoothie recipes.

John and I have learned through personal experience that proper cleansing of the organs of elimination can happen only through specific plans designed to promote "housecleaning" in each organ. We've completed numerous cleansing programs and have seen encouraging results each time. If you're ill or if you're highly motivated and have the time, you can go directly from one cleanse to the next. Alternatively, you can pace yourself with one cleanse at a time, with a break in between.

If you work away from home, you can still do the cleanse programs. Countless people have completed specific cleanses and short juice fasts and were still able to work outside their homes and even enjoy a social life. It takes some planning and preparation before each day so you can take what you need to work. You can also plan for certain social events by eating ahead of time and ordering sparkling water with lemon or lime or herbal tea at the event. You can choose what will work for you at restaurants by asking the chef to prepare all-vegetable salads or vegetable or vegan dishes. The goal is to fit the detox programs into your busy lifestyle and make them work. If you have a demanding or stressful job and you can try only one cleanse program when you have a few days off or a one-day vegetable-juice fast on a weekend day, this is a good start. Whatever positive changes you make will move you toward better health and give your overworked systems of elimination a much-needed rest so they can cleanse and rejuvenate.

# A Healthier, More Vibrant Life Awaits You

When you complete these juicing, fasting, and cleansing programs, you'll have changed your internal environment. You should feel lighter, healthier, and happier. And as a friend of mine said recently, "You'll feel like smiling all the time!" You'll have more energy to enjoy each and every day. And you'll have the best chance of preventing common and even serious illnesses. If you're ill, you'll give your body the greatest chance to heal. Best of all, you'll have discovered a way of life that will help you feel and look alive and vibrant each and every day. As my friend and popular talk show host Dr. Alvin Jones said, you feel "born again." A healthier, more balanced life truly does await you!

# CHAPTER ONE

## The Secrets of Vibrant Health

Healthy, trim, energetic, and full of life! That's what you can be when you incorporate the secrets of juicing, fasting, and cleansing, along with more raw, whole, organic foods into your lifestyle. You can easily make these wonderful steps to healing and vitality a part of your daily life. You're about to discover a program that really works. It's worked for us and for thousands of other people. It can work for you.

If you're feeling sick and tired much of the time despite your best efforts at living a healthy life, don't be discouraged. I'll help you turn that around. Maybe you've been struggling to lose weight and just can't seem to get it off or keep it off—you lose a few pounds only to gain them back, plus a few more. Or maybe you're feeling sluggish and tired; fatigue is a constant reminder that something's amiss. Perhaps you have frequent headaches, back pain, or pain elsewhere in your body. Your sleep may be disturbed; you may wake up around three a.m. each night (a good indication that you need to do a liver cleanse). Or you may feel tired in the morning, even after plenty of sleep. Your digestion may be off-kilter—you experience gas, bloating, or constipation, good indicators that you need liver and gallbladder cleansing. Your immune system may not be up to par, and consequently you experience frequent colds, flu, infections, or sinus problems. (Sinus problems may also be caused by a congested liver.) All these symptoms could be signals that your body is in need of the super nutrition found in fresh juice and the detox programs on these pages.

Whatever your health challenges or goals may be, you can benefit from the life-giving nutrients in freshly made juice and raw foods. You can get an energy and vitality boost from short juice fasts. And, because your system may be overloaded and overworked trying to clear out excess toxicity that has accumulated in your cells, tissues, and organs, you could greatly benefit from the detox programs in *Juicing, Fasting, and Detoxing for Life.*

## Detoxing for Radiant Health

Research shows that the average person is exposed to thousands of toxins and environmental pollutants daily, more than ever before in history, and all this toxic waste takes a toll on the body. Without a periodic program of detoxing, it's almost impossible to stay on top of eliminating all this stuff and keep your body in a state of health. But take heart. I'll show you how to use juicing, fasting, and detoxing programs to systematically clean out your cells, tissues, and organs of elimination and jump-start your health right away.

Detox programs and products are showing up nearly everywhere these days as people discover how they improve health. Plus, a lot of people simply feel they are toxic and in need of help. There are books and magazines that continue to promote the newest detox plans. Numerous health spas offer special detox wraps, massages, and natural mineral springs (which promote detox). There are numerous retreats and programs that offer juice fasts, raw foods, and cleansing programs to revamp your health and vitality. Health food stores have huge displays of cleansing and detox products. And it seems that nearly everyone we talk to about detoxing has an opinion or a question about how to do it or how it will be of benefit to them.

Unfortunately, many products and plans either don't work or are difficult to use. Some of the programs require little or no effort on your part; they say just take the pills or herbal products or try this quick-fix treatment and you're done—your nagging symptoms will all disappear. Keep in mind that there are no quick fixes. It took a number of years to get to this point, and it will take awhile to get your health cleared up. But while it requires time, patience, and some discipline, it's not difficult. And the rewards are huge.

Many people tell me they eat a reasonably healthy diet, get some exercise regularly, and don't eat bad stuff like junk food or desserts—at least not too often. Some people ask,

"But isn't it good enough just to eat lots of fruits and vegetables, drink some vegetable juice, buy organic produce most of the time, and try not to eat too much junk?" That's a fair maintenance program, but that's not going to clean out toxins stored in the body.

I got a call one day from a lady looking for help for her husband, who had just been diagnosed with cancer. They had been on a health regimen for more than eight years, juicing, making green smoothies, eating organic foods, exercising faithfully, and walking nearly every day. Then her husband was diagnosed with cancer. "What happened?" she asked. My first thought was to ask if he had been exposed to any toxic chemicals. He had— very potent chemicals on his job. There was the key. Just juicing and eating good foods won't clear from the body all the toxic chemicals that can be stored in organs, tissues, and fluids.

To get rid of toxins and keep your body healthy, you need to detox it periodically. That doesn't happen when you're eating regular meals all the time. Your body has to concentrate on digestion all day long. Consequently, it doesn't have much time for cleanup and repair, let alone time to move out toxins that are tucked away in fat cells, organs, and tissue spaces. To accomplish detoxification, you need to juice fast once in a while and utilize the colon, liver and gallbladder, and kidney cleanses periodically. This is the best way to stay trim, fit, and healthy or to get well again. And it's possible to accomplish this in the real world without being overly obsessed. It can even be fun once you get the hang of it.

Periodic detoxing can help you get rid of irritating toxins

that do harm in the body and stubborn fat like belly fat. The key word here is "periodic." I'm not telling you to live on only juices, raw foods, and herbs for the rest of your life, but to periodically detoxify your body with the programs in this book, to juice most days of the week, and to eat a high percentage of your food raw. Once you've completed a detox program, you can follow up with a maintenance program of whole foods, plenty of fresh vegetable juices, raw foods, purified water, regular exercise, and emotional and spiritual cleansing. I'll show you how to make it work no matter how busy or complicated your life might be. And if you're short on funds, I've got many programs you can put together inexpensively.

Since it's nearly impossible to meet your health and wellness goals without doing something to counteract the influences of ever-increasing toxicity, whether it's physical, emotional, mental, or spiritual, you must tackle the negativity with determination. Nevertheless, you don't want to be compulsively regimented about food and dieting, or anything else for that matter. I'm not advocating overdoing it to the point of making your eating habits a source of stress or fear, which will only make you feel worse, because you're probably already trying to fit a lot into your busy life. Some people tend to go overboard on health and dieting. They become food police for themselves and others, frequently driving themselves into a state of stress and exhaustion in their pursuit of perfect health. This can undo all the hard work of getting healthy. The point of this book is to guide you toward a balanced lifestyle, by making juicing a way of life, helping you find short-term cleansing programs that work for you, and providing useful tips, delicious recipes, and support to keep you on track along the way.

## Why You Need to Detox

Even if you moved to a deserted island in the middle of the South Pacific and ate only organic coconuts and vegetables grown in your own garden, you still could not be sure you were totally safe from pollution. The air you breathe might have picked up radiation from halfway around the globe; the fish you caught could be contaminated with mercury from a far-off shore; the water might not be safe to drink due to acid rain.

The reality is that we live on a planet that is polluted. The air we breathe is loaded with invisible pollutants, our food supplies are often toxic due to pesticides and preservatives, and we can't trust the water supply due to water-treatment chemicals. We are exposed to thousands of toxins and chemicals in our homes, yards, workplaces, and schools, on our highways, where we shop, in our sleep, and in the food we eat. It doesn't matter how old we are, what we do for a living, or even where we live. Environmental pollution is everywhere. These toxins include industrial chemicals, insecticides, pesticides, heavy metals, emissions from the burning of organic fuels, electromagnetic pollution, radiation, hormones and antibiotics used in animal farming, and food dyes, preservatives, and additives added to our food. We're bombarded with reactive molecules called free radicals that can damage our cells. The use of pharmaceutical and over-the-counter drugs results in side effects; moreover, these drugs can interact with other drugs and substances to cause further toxicity. Average people like you and me are being inundated with thousands of chemicals whose names most of us can't pronounce and that are invisible to us, yet inevitably they take a toll on our bodies. The assault on our bodies continues year after year, gradually weakening our organs and compromising our immune systems—our bodies' natural defense.

Toxic chemicals affect every aspect of our bodies in some way—cells, tissues, and organs become overloaded with waste. Fortunately, we are equipped with organs of elimination and detoxification to clear away the accumulation of these pollutants. But when our organs become overwhelmed with too much work, a buildup of toxicity occurs and we become more and more fatigued, mentally fogged, and susceptible to sickness. *Juicing, Fasting, and Detoxing for Life* shows you what you can do to assist your body in managing this onslaught from the environment and how to choose good health habits that will strengthen and protect you. A strong, healthy body can resist toxic overload and disease, so there's great incentive to become stronger, healthier, and more resistant.

## Some Startling Effects of Toxicity

Many studies and reports link environmental pollution to the state of our health. Chemicals that were designed to enhance our lives were introduced into our environment more than fifty years ago, but in the past half century hundreds of them have been shown to be either highly toxic and carcinogenic, or at least troublesome and irritating to our complex biological systems. It leaves us wondering what happened between what was supposed to make our lives better and what is instead making us sick.

Less than 10 percent of all the chemicals in our environment have been even partially evaluated for safety. It's difficult to know exactly how many of them are actually harmful or highly carcinogenic and could damage our health, the health of our children, and the health of our planet. Environmental toxins disrupt normal metabolic functioning of the body, which over time can lead to poor quality of life, and have been linked to conditions such as chronic fatigue syndrome, fibromyalgia, autoimmune disorders, inflammatory diseases, infertility, sexual development abnormalities, and cancer.

## Better Choices for Better Health

Now that we recognize that we live in a polluted world, what can we do to protect ourselves against this onslaught? Obviously, the first line of defense is to avoid toxins as much as possible and build up our immune systems. Although we can't avoid all exposure to environmental chemicals, especially those that we breathe, we do have many and varied choices about what we put in our mouths and on our bodies, spray in our houses and on our lawns, use for cleaning products, and apply as cosmetics.

When it comes to water, we can use purified for drinking and food preparation in order to avoid the hidden sources of pollution. Make sure to use purified water for soup, coffee, tea, and ice cubes as well. And healthy food choices are something we can make each and every day. We can choose whole, unprocessed, organic foods grown without pesticides and chemical fertilizers. When choosing animal products, we can look for cage-free eggs and cage-free poultry and grass-fed beef, raised without hormones and antibiotics.

"What am I supposed to do?" a friend asked in frustration. "If the world is so toxic and there is no escape, why even try? Maybe I should just eat all the hamburgers, French fries, and chocolate chip cookies I want!" Well, that's certainly not the answer. We can make good choices and avoid some of the more flagrant sources of poisons, such as junk food, fried food, refined carbs, high-fat and high-sugar foods, and packaged items with preservatives. We can avoid pesticides and insecticides from nonorganic foods and from those that are made for home and garden. We can say no to vaccinations, some of which still contain thimerosal, a mercury-containing organic compound that is widely used as a preservative in a number of biological and drug products, including vaccines. (This preservative could be especially harmful for babies and children and has been linked to autism, though this link is unproven. Before you get any vaccinations for yourself or your children, make sure they contain no thimerosal or any other harmful preservatives. Why be a test case for a mercury-based product?) We can avoid mercury toxicity by asking our dentists to remove all amalgam fillings (silver-colored fillings containing mercury) and replace them with safer alternatives.

The use of pharmaceutical drugs often causes side effects that are worse than the conditions the drugs are designed to treat. This requires additional drugs to counteract the negative side effects of the first one, further taxing our bodies. We can get second opinions from doctors who specialize in natural medicine and search for nontoxic natural remedies whenever possible. We can also be very thoughtful about the use of over-the-counter drugs and search out natural remedies first. Although over-the-counter drugs are widely used, they present another source of toxicity.

## How Toxic Are You?

Here is a quiz you can take to find out how toxic your environment is and how toxic you may be:

| QUESTIONS | ANSWERS | POINTS |
|---|---|---|
| 1. Do you currently smoke? | yes/no | 5 |
| 2. Have you been a smoker for more than three years? | yes/no | 3 |
| 3. Do you have silver mercury fillings? | yes/no | 4 |
| 4. Do you regularly use household chemicals for cleaning, disinfecting, deodorizing, carpet cleaning, oven cleaning, stain removal? | yes/no | 2 |

5.  Have you had a root canal?           yes/no    3
6.  Do you drink unfiltered water?        yes/no    2
7.  Do you live in an urban
    environment?                         yes/no    3
8.  Do you consume alcohol?              yes/no    3
9.  Do you use antiperspirants,
    nonorganic cosmetics, skin care
    products, or hair dye?               yes/no    2 (ea)

*HAVE YOU EVER LIVED:*

10. within ten miles of a nuclear
    power plant?                         yes/no    4
11. within five miles of a toxic
    waste dump?                          yes/no    5
12. near a farm where aerial
    pesticides are used?                 yes/no    5
13. on a farm where pesticides
    are sprayed?                         yes/no    5

14. Do you have asbestos in your
    house, workplace, or school?         yes/no    3
15. Do you consume fast foods?           yes/no    2
16. Have you ever worked
    professionally with pesticides
    or chemicals?                        yes/no    5
17. Do you use pesticides on your
    residential lawn or garden?          yes/no    3
18. Do you have your clothes cleaned
    with professional dry cleaning?      yes/no    1

*(Continued)*

| QUESTIONS | ANSWERS | POINTS |
|---|---|---|
| 19. Has your home been treated for termites in the past ten years? | yes/no | 1 |
| 20. Do you consume nonorganically grown fruits and vegetables? | yes/no | 2 |
| 21. Do you live in an area where the ground is known to contain radon gas? | yes/no | 3 |
| 22. Do you eat in restaurants more than twice a week? | yes/no | 2 |
| 23. Do you have wall-to-wall carpeting (unless nontoxic)? | yes/no | 2 |
| 24. Do you cook food in a microwave oven? In nonstick pans? | yes/no | 2 each |
| 25. Do you spend less than fifteen minutes outdoors each day? | yes/no | 2 |
| 26. Do you have an energy-efficient house that rarely gets fresh air within? | yes/no | 2 |
| 27. Do you travel by air at least once a month? | yes/no | 2 |

*DO YOU EXHIBIT ANY OF THE FOLLOWING SYMPTOMS?:*

| | | |
|---|---|---|
| 28. feel fatigued for no apparent reason | yes/no | 2 |
| 29. feel lifeless, depressed | yes/no | 2 |
| 30. feel light-headed from time to time | yes/no | 1 |
| 31. have difficulty thinking clearly | yes/no | 1 |
| 32. suffer from aches and pains for no apparent reason | yes/no | 3 |
| 33. occasionally feel irritable for no reason | yes/no | 2 |

| | | | |
|---|---|---|---|
| 34. | sometimes feel anxious for no reason | yes/no | 2 |
| 35. | sometimes experience shortness of breath for no apparent reason | yes/no | 2 |

*HAVE YOU TAKEN ANY OF THE FOLLOWING DRUGS?*
*(I POINT FOR LOW USAGE; 3 POINTS FOR HIGH USAGE):*

| | | | |
|---|---|---|---|
| 36. | prescription drugs | yes/no | 1–3 |
| 37. | painkillers/tranquilizers | yes/no | 1–3 |
| 38. | psychiatric drugs | yes/no | 1–3 |
| 39. | Ritalin | yes/no | 1–3 |
| 40. | over-the-counter drugs (aspirin, etc.) | yes/no | 1–3 |
| 41. | LSD | yes/no | 1–3 |
| 42. | heroin | yes/no | 1–3 |
| 43. | cocaine | yes/no | 1–3 |
| 44. | pot | yes/no | 1–3 |
| 45. | PCP | yes/no | 1–3 |
| 46. | methadone | yes/no | 1–3 |
| 47. | steroids | yes/no | 1–3 |

*Score:*

Sum up the points for the questions that you answered with "yes". (Note: points are accumulated only for yes answers.)

| | |
|---|---|
| 1 to 15 points | You may have a low level of toxicity in your body. |
| 16 to 25 points | You may have levels of toxicity in your body that could reduce your ability to stay healthy and think clearly. |
| 26 to 40 points | You may have a level of toxicity in your body that often causes you to feel fatigued, lethargic, |

*(Continued)*

or mentally foggy or to be susceptible to colds and flu.

41 to 50 points    You may have a high level of toxicity in your body that often causes you to get sick, to feel mentally foggy, lethargic, and fatigued, to experience aches and pains, and to be susceptible to disease.

>50 points    You could be experiencing extreme body toxicity, which could include all the symptoms listed above, make you susceptible to serious disease such as cancer, and reduce the length and quality of your life.

If you scored even a few points on this quiz, this is an indication that you could benefit from cleansing your body.

### Symptoms of Toxic Overload

- Anxiety, fear, or nervousness
- Arthritis, painful joints
- Asthma or bronchitis
- Bloating or gas
- Cellulite
- Clogged sinuses
- Confusion or poor concentration
- Congestion
- Constipation
- Dark-colored, cloudy, strong-smelling urine
- Depression
- Frequent colds and flu
- Headaches

- Heartburn or indigestion
- Hives, rashes, eczema, or dry skin
- Lethargy, tiredness, or fatigue
- Mood swings
- Nausea
- Pimples or rashes
- Puffiness or dark circles under the eyes
- Runny nose or constant sneezing
- Shortness of breath
- Sleeplessness
- Water retention

## What Happens When Toxicity Builds Up?

Most of us keep our floors swept and our clothes washed, and give our cars periodic oil changes. We understand the importance of cleaning and caring for our possessions, but we often neglect our own bodies. Our bodies are able to handle a certain amount of toxicity because we have immune systems and organs of elimination designed to clean out many of these toxic substances, but they can handle only so much before they become overwhelmed by the huge numbers of toxins that we encounter from the environment—air, water, and food.

The result is that substances not broken down and excreted are generally stored in the intestines, gallbladder, kidneys, liver, lymph, fat cells, and skin. The colon, which is designed to eliminate solid waste, can become sluggish and build up putrefaction. The liver can get congested and be unable to properly filter the blood. The kidneys can become overwhelmed in their attempt to excrete toxin-laden urea. As a result, our systems are unable to function properly; nutrients are not absorbed well and poisons are reabsorbed into our bloodstreams. Toxins are then stored in fat cells, they collect in other tissues and spaces between the cells, and they clog our lymphatic systems. If the lymph isn't moving the debris out of our bodies, we can begin to feel sick. All this toxic buildup eventually affects our energy, mood, sleep, mental clarity, and immune function. We may feel sick, tired, and depressed. If we continue in this decline, we may get a disease.

## What Detoxing Will Do for You

"Detoxifying" is another word for "cleansing," which means to eliminate toxins. I'll use the words interchangeably. When you embark on a detox program, it may take some work at first, but the benefits are so astounding that the effort is worthwhile. You'll not only feel stronger and more energetic as a result; you'll start looking younger and more vibrant. You may look in the mirror one day and see fewer wrinkles and softer skin or you may notice that dark circles or puffiness under your eyes is gone. Your skin will develop an underlying glow. Your hair will shine more and become healthier and your nails will grow stronger.

People who have followed my detox programs also report greater mental clarity. "I can think straight again!" one client exclaimed. In most people there is a restored sense of well-being that may have eluded them for years. One friend said she reported to her doctor that she could never remember having a sense of well-being. His answer was to prescribe an antidepressant drug, which she refused. When I taught her about juicing, detoxing, and a whole foods diet, she reported back in a few weeks that she had finally gained that elusive sense of well-being she'd only read about.

When we give our bodies a rest from processing all the excesses, they're able to rebuild, repair, and strengthen organs and systems, which will protect us from disease. We won't be subject to every cold and flu that circulates, and our bodies can begin to heal from ailments that may have plagued us for years. Over the years I've received countless testimonies from people who have healed their bodies by juicing, fasting, and detoxing. One lady cleared up liver problems in one week with the liver cleanse. I've heard from people who have improved or healed a wide variety of ailments, from fibromyalgia to Lyme disease to cancer, with the programs in *Juicing, Fasting, and Detoxing for Life.*

Detoxing also helps us lose weight. Vast amounts of toxic substances found in our environment, including carcinogens, are stored in fat cells. Because the body uses fat to hold toxins, thereby protecting our delicate organs, we often find it hard to lose weight. Ironically, fat is our friend when it comes to toxins. It protects us from all the acidic and toxic waste that endangers our organs. But when we remove this mess through detoxing, our bodies no longer need this protection, so they can begin to let go of the extra fat. We suddenly notice that our clothes fit better and we feel lighter and happier, while fat just seems to be melting away.

## Juicing and Fasting: The Best Ways to Begin Detoxing

As you prepare to juice fast and detox, your first step is to add fresh vegetable juices that will help you transition to a healthier diet. The juices will build your body's nutritional reserves and strengthen your immune system. They'll begin to gently detox your body because they are rich in antioxidants that bind to toxins and carry them out of your system. And they prepare your body for more intense cleansing in the form of short juice fasts and detox plans. Juicing can be fun and easy, and the health results are astounding. In chapter two, I'll show you how to incorporate juicing into your busy lifestyle and make sure you look forward to every juice, smoothie, or cold soup you make. And I'll tell you which juicers are best and why. You can learn how to prepare juices quickly and easily and make delicious, nutritious juice.

The recipes in this book use very little fruit juice. Instead I focus on vegetable juicing, and raw, blended vegetable soups and green smoothies. I show you how to make the juices, smoothies, and soups taste great with additions like lemon or lime, gingerroot, or a little low-sugar fruit such as a green apple, but without the taste of sweeter fruit, while you retrain your taste buds for a whole new juicing experience. Because vegetable juices are alkalizing, they help the body flush away accumulated acids and enable it to reach a more balanced pH so it can cleanse, heal, and get rid of excess weight and cellulite. Almost all toxins are acidic, which is the opposite of alkaline, so drinking lots of vegetable juice, especially plenty of green juices, helps counteract this acidity.

Most juice books, including my first juice book, *Juicing for Life*, use too much fruit juice, which contains too much sugar. Fruit contains a lot of natural sugar, which is fine for most people when combined with insoluble and soluble fiber. (Fiber slows down sugar absorption.) But when fruit is juiced, the insoluble fiber is removed, and the fruit sugar is easily absorbed. That's why I recommend that you eat your fruit as a general rule, with the exception of low-sugar fruit such as lemon, lime, grapefruit, berries, and green apple, and juice and eat your vegetables.

For an additional health boost, I advocate adding a short juice fast for one or two days as a great way to jump-start your health or weight loss. This will give your digestive system a rest so it can process and eliminate food and waste that have accumulated over time. Juices are easy to digest and provide concentrated nutrition for energy, plus plenty of vitamins, minerals, enzymes, phytonutrients, and anti-oxidants. No matter what else you're doing, adding short vegetable-juice fasts occasionally into your diet will help you feel healthier and more energetic right away.

## Take the First Steps to a Healthy Lifestyle

The very first step in a healthy lifestyle is choosing the best food and beverages. Once you've finished the detox programs, you can maintain the ground you've gained by continuing with a diet that is based on health-building fresh vegetable juices, raw foods (50 to 75 percent of your diet), and whole, organic foods.

Most people find that once they've tried my juice recipes and completed some of the detox programs, their tastes actually change. The old, unhealthy foods they once loved no longer taste as good. They find themselves craving fresh vegetables, juices, and big green salads instead of sugary snacks or salty chips. They might enjoy an occasional meal of their old fare or a few fattening favorites, but for the most part, they want to eat foods that are fresh, whole, and natural. Once you've made some healthy changes, you should no longer crave the things that have been undermining your health and making you feel less vibrant and well.

Following are the basic components of a healthy lifestyle:

## Basics of an Alkaline Diet: Why It Matters

The tissues and organs of our bodies do best if they are sustained at a more alkaline rather than acidic pH environment. The term "pH" refers to the level of acidity and alkalinity in any environment. Battery acid is an example of a strong acid. Lye, or sodium hydroxide, is an example of a strongly alkaline substance. Water, specifically distilled water, is neutral. The pH scale goes from one to fourteen, with one being most acid, seven being neutral, and fourteen being most alkaline, or basic. Biological systems like the human body must maintain a balance in the middle range of this pH scale—between 4.0 and 9.5. Most systems, with the exception of parts of the digestive tract, function best if they are slightly alkaline; for example, saliva should be between 6.5 and 7.5 and urine should be about 7. (You can purchase pH testing strips at your pharmacy and find out just how balanced your system is.)

The typical American diet consists of an abundance of foods that create high levels of acidity in the body once they are metabolized, or broken down during digestion. Foods that are broken down to acidic residue are meats, poultry, cheese and other dairy products, fried foods, sugar of all kinds, refined flour products including pastas and breads, soft drinks, coffee, tea, beer, wine, liquor, some fruits, and all junk food. Foods that are alkaline are vegetables, vegetable juices, good oils like coconut oil and olive oil, some nuts, and most legumes.

If most of the food we eat metabolizes into an alkaline ash, it nourishes and strengthens the body and gives us plenty of energy. On the other hand, if the majority of our food is metabolized into an acidic residue, this is toxic and leads to stress on our delicate organs and tissues. Other factors also contribute to acidity, such as chemical and environmental pollutants, free radicals, and electromagnetic fields, as well as negative thoughts and emotions like fear, worry, anger, and anxiety.

### Acid Versus Alkaline Foods

**ACID**

- Coffee, tea, soda, and alcohol
- Coffee creamers
- Dairy products
- Fast foods and junk food
- Grains (bread and pasta)
- Meats and animal products
- Most fruit
- Sugar

**ALKALINE**

- Alkaline water
- Good oils (coconut oil and olive oil)
- Nuts and seeds
- Most legumes
- Some fruit
- Vegetables and vegetable juices

If our cells, tissues, and organs are fed with acidic fluids (due to poor lifestyle choices), they can become inflamed,
which can lead to diseases such as obesity, heart disease, and
cancer. Our blood is especially sensitive to pH changes. It
must maintain a level that is slightly alkaline, between 7.35
and 7.45. It's a lot like the body's temperature—too high or
too low and we can die; slightly off and we feel sick. In the
same way, if the blood becomes too acidic or too basic, we
feel sick; if it's way off, we can be in a perilous situation.

To rectify imbalances and reduce acid levels, which is
the imbalance most of us deal with, the body attempts to
neutralize acids by dumping alkaline buffers into the bloodstream. The principal buffers that react as neutralizers are
calcium phosphate and calcium carbonate, and when they
are not present from dietary supply, they're taken from our
bones. This may account for why so many women, and even
older men, are experiencing osteopenia or osteoporosis. If
we are overconsuming acidic foods, our bones become weak
and porous. Also, in an acidic environment, we can easily
develop painful joints and arthritis, even joint deterioration
as in osteoarthritis and degenerative hip-joint disease. Our
organs and other tissues suffer from inflammation caused
by the acidity and shortage of minerals to help neutralize it.
An overly acidic body is also a toxic body. Microorganisms
like bacteria, viruses, fungus, and yeast thrive in an acidic
medium, as do cancer cells, but they do not thrive in an alkaline balanced environment.

Too much acidity also can cause us to gain weight or prevent us from losing weight. The body tends to store acid in fat cells and hang on to the fat to keep the acidity from doing more damage in other areas of the body. Often, when people bring their bodies into a healthy pH balance, the weight seems to just melt off.

You can best maintain a proper pH by balancing your diet with 50 to 75 percent alkaline foods and juices, along with pure water (alkaline water is even better), exercise, and positive thoughts and emotions. You can still enjoy some of your favorite acid-forming foods if you make them no more than 25 to 30 percent of your diet.

## Good Fats and Oils

It's essential in any healthy dietary program to include plenty of good fats and oils. Many people still think that a low-fat diet is the only way to stay slim and maintain health, especially heart health, but current research has shown that a low-fat diet is unhealthy and points to the importance of providing plenty of essential fatty acids and other good fats.

For several decades we have been inundated with advertising that promotes vegetable oils like safflower, sunflower, soy, corn, and canola oil. However, these oils are all made up of long-chain fatty acids (LCFAs), which contribute to weight gain because the body tends to store them rather than burn them. These oils have also been implicated as contributors to heart disease and other health problems because they oxidize easily (meaning they react with oxygen, for example, and form an oxide). It is oxidized cholesterol that is harmful, not normal cholesterol. When heated, vegetable oils oxidize and can cause free-radical damage; at high heat they form trans fats, which generate even more free radicals, which cause myriad health problems, including heart disease. Once a free-radical reaction is started, it can create a chain reaction, which produces more free radicals and can ultimately damage thousands of molecules.

One of the classic signs of old age is the appearance of brown, freckle-like spots known as liver spots or sunspots. They are signs of free-radical deterioration in the lipids (fats) in our skin, thus the name *lipo*fuscin. Oxidation of polyunsaturated fats and protein by free-radical activity in the skin is recognized as one of the major causes of liver spots, along with liver congestion and toxicity. Liver spots don't ordinarily cause physical discomfort, but they do affect our appearance, and that can cause emotional discontent. They are a result of internal reactions that can undermine our health. Because cells cannot dispose of the lipofuscin pigment, it gradually accumulates within many cells of the body as we age. Once lipofuscin pigment develops, it tends to stick around for life, but you can prevent further oxidation, and perhaps even reduce the spots you already have, by using the right kinds of oils in your diet and on your skin.

I recommend virgin coconut oil and extra-virgin olive oil as the best oils for food preparation and cosmetic use. Coconut oil is made up of primarily medium-chain triglycerides (MCTs). The liver especially likes to burn the MCTs in coconut oil, which means this oil will help you lose weight. MCTs act more like kindling in a fire than like a big log. Other oils, made up of long-chain triglycerides (LCTs), contribute to weight gain because the body tends to store them rather than burn them. They are the body's "big logs in the fireplace." They are also easily oxidized, as already discussed. Take a look at our book *The Coconut Diet* for the Coconut Diet weight-loss program, which has helped thousands of people lose weight and feel healthier. It offers a full discussion of the benefits of coconut oil and how it compares to other oils, along with information on how to use it in more than seventy delicious recipes.

Olive oil is heart healthy and part of the Mediterranean diet. Olive oil is called virgin if it is extracted by means of pressure from millstones. The first pressing is the most flavorful and has the least acidity; it's called extra virgin. The first cold pressing also has the highest amount of fatty acids and polyphenols (antioxidants). Olive oils from the Mediterranean, and particularly Spain, are the highest in antioxidants. The very best choice is extra-virgin, cold-pressed olive oil that is organically grown in the Mediterranean.

## Water and the Importance of Hydrating

Our bodies are more than 70 percent water, so we need to continually drink purified water to keep properly hydrated. Water is vital to health because it helps flush waste through the system. If you're dehydrated, you can become constipated,

acidic, and fatigued. We depend on water for our very exis-
tence, yet many people simply do not drink enough water, or
enough of the right type of water. Fortunately it has become
somewhat fashionable to carry water bottles wherever we go,
and the educated public is beginning to understand the importance of drinking water. Still, if you ask the average person
how much water he or she drinks, that person will probably
tell you one or two pint bottles a day. Some people say they
don't even like water and refuse to drink it. However, at least
eight to ten 8-ounce glasses of water a day (2 to 2 1/2 quarts) is
recommended for good health. If you are detoxing, are a large
person, or are very active, 3 to 4 quarts a day is optimum.

Water increases endurance and energy, aids digestion,
regulates body temperature, and facilitates muscular and
nervous system activity. Our bodies are designed to deliver
essential nutrients, oxygen, hormones, and antibodies into
our cells through an aqueous medium. When the body is
properly hydrated, it's able to deliver nutrients and remove
toxic waste products that have been accumulating over time.

The water from most kitchen taps is generally not good
for drinking. As it travels through the many miles of pipe
(many of them in our cities are very old and some are deterio-
rating) and earth, it picks up thousands of microscopic impurities such as pesticides, industrial chemicals, heavy metals,
parasites, and other toxins. Most city tap water has added
chemicals like chlorine and fluoride, which are also harmful
to our bodies. Therefore, it's vitally important that we drink
the purest water possible.

### Filter Your Water

Most tap water in the United States contains fluoride, a toxic industrial chemical that has been widely promoted as being healthy for the public. In reality, however, fluoride is a poison that may harm your health. Did you know?

- Fluoride is a toxic industrial waste product, which may be contaminated with lead, arsenic, radionucleotides, aluminum, and other industrial contaminants. Fluoride that is added to municipal water supplies is not pharmaceutical grade.
- Twenty-three studies from four countries show that even moderate exposure to fluoride lowers IQ.
- The daily fluoride dose recommended by the American Dental Association results in the same level of fluoride in your blood shown to cause an 8-point drop in IQ.
- You should call poison control if you swallow a quarter milligram of fluoride from toothpaste; however, one glass of water can contain this amount of fluoride.
- To remain within "safe" limits, you'd have to use such a small amount of fluoridated toothpaste that one tube would last for several years.

When it comes to purified water, there are several options: distillers, sediment filters, activated carbon filters, kinetic degradation fluxion filters, and reverse osmosis. There are water filtration systems that also ionize the water, thus enabling you to set the controls to produce alkaline water, which is a huge plus in keeping your system in alkaline balance. But always make sure that the filter system you purchase also removes fluoride. It is a tough chemical to remove, and some filter systems need a special attachment to remove it.

Whatever you do, avoid bottled water in #7 plastic bottles.

A number is required on all plastic so you can determine what kind of plastic is used, and #7 is used for almost all plastic water bottles, including the five-gallon bottles for home and office coolers. This plastic used for bottles and many plastic food containers includes phthalates, which are compounds used in inks, adhesives, vinyl floor tiles, and paints. They make plastic more flexible, but they're troublesome because they leach into the water or food being stored. They have the potential to cause male offspring to be more feminine and develop small or abnormal reproductive organs, and are associated with early puberty in girls and miscarriages in women. Women who are pregnant or planning on getting pregnant should especially avoid water from #7 plastic bottles and #7 plastic food containers. (Look for the number imprinted on the container or bottle, usually on the bottom.)

You can opt for safer choices for water bottles and food and beverage storage, which includes polypropylene (#5 PP), high-density polyethylene (#2 HDPE), and low-density polyethylene (#4 LDPE). Still, all plastic does leach some toxins into the water or food. (It is believed that the only way to get rid of plastic toxins is to do the sauna detox program.)

For transporting water, you can purchase nontoxic water bottles that don't leach phthalates or aluminum and don't harbor bacteria. There are many stainless steel water bottles available. (Go to your health food store or online and you'll find many websites that sell nontoxic water bottles.)

### Dangerous Chemical Found in Plastic

According to a statement by several dozen scientists, as well as reports from federal health agencies, an estrogen-like compound widely used in plastic products is thought to be causing serious reproductive disorders. The compound is bisphenol A (BPA) and is one of the most-produced chemicals in the world. Almost everyone has traces of it in their bodies. A new study by the National Institutes of Health found that newborn animals exposed to BPA suffered from uterine damage. The damage could indicate that this chemical causes reproductive disorders in women ranging from fibroids to endometriosis to cancer.

After reviewing nearly seven hundred studies, scientists concluded that people are exposed to levels of BPA in excess of those that have harmed lab animals. Among the most vulnerable are infants and fetuses that are still developing. BPA is used to make hard plastic that's used in numerous products, including:

- Polycarbonate plastic baby bottles
- Large water-cooler containers and sports bottles
- Microwave-oven dishes
- Canned-food liners
- Some dental sealants for children

Problems associated with even small amounts of BPA include:

- Structural damage to the brain
- Hyperactivity
- Abnormal sexual behavior
- Increased fat formation and risk of obesity
- Early puberty and disrupted reproductive cycles

#### Ten Tips to Reduce Your Exposure to BPA

1. Use only glass baby bottles and dishes for your baby.
2. Give your baby natural fabric toys instead of plastic ones.
3. Store your food and beverages in glass—not plastic—containers.
4. Avoid using a microwave as much as possible, but if you do, don't microwave food in a plastic container.
5. Completely avoid canned foods and drinks.
6. Avoid using plastic wrap (and never microwave anything covered in it).

*(Continued)*

7. Get rid of plastic dishes, glasses, and cups, and replace them with glass.
8. If you opt to use plastic kitchenware, at least get rid of the older, scratched-up varieties, avoid putting them in the dishwasher, and don't wash them with harsh detergents, as these things can cause more chemicals to leach into your food. In the event that you do opt to use plastic containers for your food, be sure to avoid those marked on the bottom with the recycling label #7, as these varieties may contain BPA.
9. Avoid using bottled water; filter your own instead.
10. Before allowing a dental sealant to be applied to your teeth or to your children's, ask your dentist to verify that it does not contain BPA. Also, don't allow fluoride to be applied to teeth.

## The Value of Eating Whole Foods

Whole foods are foods that are unprocessed and unrefined, or processed and refined as little as possible before being consumed. Modern food processing strips away nutrients and fiber and often forms harmful chemicals in the process. These alien food substances are difficult for the body to metabolize.

Often confused with organically grown food, whole foods aren't necessarily organic, nor are organic foods necessarily whole, but organic and whole are the most desirable foods to choose. Because of the lack of preservatives, many whole foods have a short shelf life, but they also have more life-giving nutrients and fewer toxins than processed food. This makes them very desirable when it comes to health.

Examples of whole foods include unpolished grains, unprocessed fruits and vegetables, and unpasteurized milk. The further away we get from the original food, the less whole it is, such as in instant potatoes versus whole potatoes, pressed turkey versus whole turkey, margarine versus butter, or vegetable oil versus the seeds or vegetables it's made from.

## Why It's Important to Eat Raw Foods

It is preferable to eat 50 to 75 percent of our whole foods raw to obtain the maximum nutritional and health-related benefits. Scientific evidence shows that raw foods have significant long-term health benefits. For example, an article published in the *Journal of Nutrition* (April 1992) shows that raw vegan diets significantly decreased LDL cholesterol and triglycerides. Other research shows that shifting from a conventional diet to predominantly foods that are uncooked can result in a decrease in bacterial enzymes and certain toxic products in the body.

So what does heat do to our food? Chemical changes take place in individual nutrients as excessive heat is applied. Excessive heat breaks down vitamins, enzymes, and amino acids, destroys biophotons, and produces undesirable cross-linkages in proteins, particularly in meat. When food is heated above 118°F for three minutes or longer, deleterious changes begin to take place and progressively cause increased nutritional damage as higher temperatures are applied over longer periods of time. For example, proteins coagulate because high temperatures denature protein molecular structure, leading to deficiency of some essential amino acids. (However, meat, poultry, and fish must be thoroughly cooked at 325°F to 350°F.) Carbohydrates caramelize, and fats oxidize and generate numerous carcinogens including acrolein, nitrosamines, hydrocarbons, and benzopyrene (one of the most potent cancer-causing agents known). Many vitamins and biophotons are destroyed and most of the enzymes are damaged. Further, the body must produce more enzymes to help digest cooked food, which drains energy needed to maintain and repair tissue and organ systems. Also, pesticides can restructure into even more toxic compounds, and free radicals are produced.

### Is Microwaving Food Harmful?

The following is a summary of a 1976 Russian investigation of microwave ovens:

- Some studies suggest microwaving your food can potentially expose you to carcinogenic toxins released from plastic or paper wrappers, destruction of valuable nutrients in the food, and radiation leakage.
- Swiss food scientist Dr. Hans Hertel found that microwaved food increased cholesterol levels, decreased both red and white blood cell counts, decreased hemoglobin, and produced radiolytic compounds.

There are many things you can do to preserve your food, such as dehydrating foods like crackers, onions, tomatoes, and even kale and Swiss chard at 118°F or below (considered raw food); they are healthful and delicious! (See the Resources Guide for dehydrator recommendations.) And you can gently warm vegetable foods (not animal products), keeping the temperature at 118°F or below, which helps preserve nutrient content.

The reasons why raw foods are so life-giving haven't

been thoroughly researched, but the experience is unmistakable. Eating more raw organic food is one of the best ways to improve your health; it builds your immune system and prevents disease. Finding ways to get more raw foods into your diet, such as juicing every day, is one of the keys to vibrant health.

---

### Making Wise Food Choices

Make these food choices a major part of your diet:

- Whole, unprocessed food
- Organically grown food
- Fresh vegetables
- Raw nuts and seeds
- Whole grains (avoid wheat; it's been too hybridized and now contains too much gluten)
- Legumes (beans, lentils, split peas)
- Whole low-sugar fruit such as green apples and berries
- Free-range poultry (in small amounts)
- Grass-fed beef (in small amounts)
- Grass-fed and free-range meats (in small amounts)
- Organic, free-range eggs
- Plenty of alkaline foods; about 70 to 75 percent of your diet
- Good fats and oils (virgin coconut oil and extra-virgin olive oil)
- Eight to ten glasses of purified water per day, stored in nontoxic water bottles
- Little or no stimulants such as coffee and black tea (green, white, and herbal teas are fine) and alcohol

---

## Exercise

Exercise is essential for a strong body and vibrant health, and it keeps us trim and fit so we look great and have plenty of energy for daily work and recreation. Exercise physiologists tell us that even short periods of exercise over time will provide enormous benefits. We will not only look and feel better; we will be nourished and strengthened—inside and out.

Daily exercise or movement of some kind is also necessary for effective internal function of our bodies. It is especially crucial during the detoxing process because the movement carries waste products out of our systems and strengthens the immune system. Regular movement also keeps the heart and cardiovascular system strong, enables the body to properly metabolize nutrients, and builds new proteins and hormones. It also helps us sleep better at night, a big plus for the cleansing, healing process.

## Emotional and Spiritual Health

Our lives are often harried and stressful. We're under pressure to do more than we have time or energy to accomplish. Negative, angry, critical, or unforgiving thoughts about ourselves and others can wreak havoc on our nervous, cardiovascular, and endocrine systems, which then affects every organ and tissue in our bodies, often translating into myriad health problems.

Even if you are eating well and exercising regularly, negative thoughts and emotions can bring about a cascading response from the endocrine system, which releases hormones like adrenaline and cortisol that lead to fight-or-flight reactions. Constant overstimulation and exposure to these stress hormones weakens our immune systems and eventu-

ally leads to diseases and biological disorders. Stress also damages the liver, which is the principal organ of detoxification in the body; it is also quite sensitive to anger. Stress and negative emotions can weaken the kidneys, which are particularly sensitive to fear, and the lungs, which are very sensitive to grief. While our bodies are healing and we are cleansing, we should care for and nurture our souls. (See chapter eight for an extensive discussion of thoughts and emotions as they relate to detoxing and to health.)

## A Pep Talk for the Juicing, Fasting, and Detoxing Programs

Some days we're just too busy or stressed out to stay on a strict program, so don't try to be perfect all the time; just do the best you can. And remember, it's still better to do something good for yourself than to lapse into totally unhealthy patterns. Ask yourself: "Is this going to make me feel better and build my health, or is it going to make me feel worse and undermine my hard work in the end?" If you're mad at yourself about a little indulgence or about getting off a cleanse program, you may slip back into some old, unhealthy patterns and just decide to blow it completely. Instead, love and forgive yourself for not being perfect. Get a little exercise, relax, drink some water or make a glass of juice, take a few deep breaths, pick up a good book, pray or meditate, spend time with friends and family, and get back in the rhythm of a healthy life. No one's perfect, but you want to feel good and care for the wonderful body you've been given so you'll have energy for work, pleasure, enjoying your friends and family, and fulfilling your purpose. Tell yourself that you can do it. You're a strong person who deserves to experience vibrant health.

**The Secrets of Vibrant Health: Summary**

- Reduce environmental toxins.
- Make wise food choices.
- Increase exercise.
- Find emotional, mental, and spiritual balance.

# CHAPTER TWO

## *Juicing for Life*

Recently, someone asked me if they couldn't just drink V8 juice and eat more salads and get the same effect as juicing fresh produce. First, most of us just can't seem to eat enough fresh vegetables each day to reach even the minimum number of servings suggested for good health. And processed juices—canned, bottled, or frozen—have had a lot of nutrients, enzymes, and biophotons destroyed in the processing, so they fall short when it comes to revitalizing the body; they are not considered live food. But probably the most compelling reason to juice is that fresh juice provides an excellent way for us to absorb vitamins and minerals, which is even superior to eating whole vegetables, because juicing releases these nutrients in a highly absorbable form. So as you embark on your journey to vibrant health, eat whole foods—at least 50 to 75 percent of them should be raw. Drink plenty of water. And juice a lot of vegetables most days of the week.

If you're wondering how you can possibly fit juicing into a schedule that is so busy you can barely get everything done in a day, I'll show you how to make it work. Some people say they're intimidated by the whole prospect of juicing, imagining it to be a daunting, messy, and time-consuming process. Others think it's so difficult that only professionals can do it right, so they never even get started. One lady told me she drove around with a juicer in the trunk of her car for two months before she had the courage to even take it inside her house. If you're among those who are confused or intimidated, I'll help you. There are dozens of tips on how to choose and use a juicer in the pages that follow. You'll be "juicing it up" in no time. And if you're still a bit confused, just go to my website, JuiceLadyCherie.com, for more information on how you can jump into juicing; then, if you still need extra help, contact me. I'll get you through the process (see the Resources Guide).

The good news is that there are many ways to make juicing quick, easy, and a regular part of your life. When you've finished this chapter, you'll see that even a beginner can have a juicer up and running in a short time. The latest juicers are designed for busy people because the manufacturers have figured out that most people won't use them unless they're easy to operate and clean. Some of the newest machines are very fast. I've timed myself and found that I can make the morning juice for my husband and myself in about ten minutes from start to finish, which includes cleanup. The actual juicing process (not counting produce prep time) is one minute with the juicer I use each day. And the cleanup time is one minute. There are juicers with super-wide feeding tubes at the top so you don't have to cut the produce into little pieces. The best ones are designed to expel the pulp into a container that you can line with a free baggie from the grocery store produce section. That way, you can just dump the whole thing in the trash or the compost pile when you're done and you don't have to wash the pulp catcher. Plus, most of the newer-model juicers are easier than ever to clean because they have only a few parts to wash and most of those are dishwasher safe.

There are also steps you can take in advance to save time. For example, you can wash and prepare your produce the night before or perhaps on the weekend to make juicing in the morning even faster. You can place your washed produce in airtight glass containers, or the new green bags that keep produce fresh longer. That way you can grab a handful of each of your favorite veggies with a bit of low-sugar fruit if you wish, toss them into the juicer, and be done juicing in a matter of minutes. (You can also make your juice the night before and store it in an airtight container in the refrigerator.) Then simply rinse off the juicer parts and place them in the upper rack of your dishwasher. It's really that easy. Either drink the juice right away or store it in an airtight container such as a thermos and be off for the day! And you can make extra juice for later. It's great to have some freshly made juice for a midmorning break at work or with lunch. Some people make a big batch of juice on the weekend and freeze it in individual containers.

It's possible—and easy—to juice up more produce in one glass than many people will eat in a day—maybe even more than you'd put in a big main-course salad. For example, on most mornings, I juice one very large cucumber, two to four carrots, a handful of parsley, two ribs of celery, a two-inch piece of gingerroot, several leaves of chard or kale, and half a lemon. I then pour the juice into the blender, add an avocado, and turn this into a green smoothie. (This serves two, and that's just our starting juice for the day.)

Once you realize how healthy and energizing it is to drink fresh juice each day, and how great you feel, I think you'll be motivated to find a way to juice up your favorite produce regularly. Whether you're a busy executive, a career mom or dad, or someone who's just always on the go, juicing will give you the energy and vitality to accomplish more and feel great while you're doing it. And you don't want to wait until you're sick, like I did, to start a health-building program. Juicing is the best fast food in the world—it provides quick energy that lasts throughout the day and will put you on the fast track to health. You'll find you just aren't as hungry so it's easier to maintain your weight. When you drink this life-giving nutrition in a glass, you're sowing great seeds of health that will serve you for years to come.

## Fresh Juice or Liquid Candy

Fresh juice prepared at home in your juicer is one of the healthiest alternatives to other popular beverages like soft drinks, which contain 10 teaspoons of sugar per 12-ounce can. But whether they're sugar-sweetened or artificially sweetened diet sodas, soft drinks contribute to obesity and a host of other health problems. That's because the massive amount of sugar they contain causes an insulin burst that turns the sugar into fat. A recent study showed that those who drink two to three regular soft drinks a day have a 35 percent greater chance of being overweight. Diet sodas are even more likely to pack on the pounds. Surprisingly, 55 percent of the people who drank two to three diet sodas per day were shown to be overweight. Diet sodas and other diet products contain artificial sweeteners that overexcite the nervous system, causing people to want more and more sweet foods. Studies showed that those who drank the most artificially sweetened beverages gained the most weight. Artificial sweeteners, such as aspartame, have been associated with brain tumors. Sucralose (Splenda) has been associated with thymus gland shrinkage.

### Components of a Can of Soda

- **Phosphoric acid** can interfere with the body's ability to use calcium, leading to osteoporosis or softening of the teeth and bones. It also neutralizes hydrochloric acid in your stomach, which can interfere with digestion, making it difficult to utilize nutrients.
- **Sugar** increases insulin levels, which can lead to high blood pressure, high cholesterol, heart disease, diabetes, weight gain, premature aging, and many more negative side effects.
- **Aspartame** is used as a sugar substitute in diet soda. There are numerous side effects associated with aspartame consumption, including brain tumors, birth defects, diabetes, emotional disorders, and epilepsy and seizures.
- **Caffeine** in drinks causes jitters, insomnia, high blood pressure, irregular heartbeat, elevated blood cholesterol levels, vitamin and mineral depletion, breast lumps, and birth defects.
- **Tap water** is the main ingredient in bottled soft drinks. It can carry numerous chemicals including chlorine, trihalomethanes, lead, cadmium, and various organic pollutants.

*(Continued)*

Sodas also contribute to toxicity. They contain artificial colorings, especially yellow dye no. 5, which has been shown to promote attention-deficit hyperactivity disorder (ADHD) in some children. Yellow dye no. 5 also causes hives, asthma, and other allergic reactions in a small number of individuals. The chemicals in sodas break down into even more toxic by-products once ingested, taxing the liver and leading to symptoms such as headaches, depression, lethargy, certain autoimmune disorders, and low thyroid function. Also, they can lead to low blood sugar, diabetes, and cravings for more sweet carbohydrates. Consumption of soft drinks may also increase the risk of osteoporosis because phosphorus, a common ingredient in soda, has been shown to deplete bones of calcium.

So when you're on the go, take fresh juice in a thermos for a healthy pick-me-up. There are also unsweetened waters with flavors such as cranberry-orange, pear, pomegranate-tangerine, and raspberry-lime. These are much healthier choices than the "liquid candy" people are downing.

Psychologists tell us it takes about twenty-one days to develop a new habit, and those twenty-one days of juicing will propel you into a whole new level of health. To help motivate you, the next section will give you an overview of the many ways juicing can build your health and energize every cell in your body. You'll also find nutritional information about what vegetable juice contains, so you'll know more about what it's doing for you. Once you see all the benefits, you just may be sold on juicing for the rest of your life.

## Why Drink Juice?

Fresh juice contains an abundance of nutrients that will energize your body, build your health, and help you fight disease. Juice provides water, easily absorbed amino acids and carbohydrates, plus a virtual cornucopia of vitamins, minerals, enzymes, antioxidants, phytonutrients, biophotons, and soluble fiber. Scientists are now showing that the phytonutrients found in plants may be even more important for our health than vitamins and minerals. Without all these life-giving substances, found principally in vegetables and fruit, our immune systems weaken and we become subject to various disturbances, which can lead to feeling sick and tired most of the time and to illness and disease.

Forget the "5 a day"! The latest nutritional guidelines show that we need between nine and thirteen servings of vegetables and fruit per day to stay healthy, depending on age and activity level, with an emphasis on leafy dark-green vegetables and red and yellow vegetables and fruit. It was hard enough to get even five of these life-giving foods in our diet each and every day. Juicing is about the only way many of us can get more. The following equals one serving: 1/2 cup of raw or cooked vegetables, 3/4 cup of vegetable juice, and 1 cup of raw leafy vegetables. So if you're going for the minimum of nine servings daily, you'll need something like 1 to 2 cups of leafy green vegetables (that's about one salad) and 4 cups of fruits and vegetables. That's not easy to do most days. Juicing can really help you fill in the gaps. When you juice a lot of veggies, eat a piece or two of fruit, have a big salad and a steamed vegetable, you'll reach the recommended goal.

There's another great benefit. Because fresh juice is loaded with antioxidants that bind to toxins and carry them out of the body so they don't damage your cells, it offers a gentle way to begin detoxifying your system. Your digestive system doesn't have to expend a lot of energy to break down juice. Therefore, it can use the energy to detoxify your body, make repairs, and build your health. Scientists are continuing to discover how various nutrients found in fresh juice build your immune system, help prevent disease, and heal specific ailments. See the following box regarding the latest research on the healing benefits of vegetables, keeping in mind that juice made from these foods makes the nutrients in them highly available to fight off diseases and build immunity.

### Scientific Research and the Healing Benefits of Vegetables and Fruit

Science has shown that a diet rich in vegetables and fruit can lower the risk and symptoms of the following diseases:

#### Cardiovascular Disease

A diet rich in vegetables and fruit has been found to lower the risk of heart disease and stroke. The most comprehensive research study to date was done by the Harvard School of Public Health. Researchers followed the health and dietary habits of 110,000 men and women for fourteen years and found that the higher the average daily intake of vegetables and fruit, the lower the chances of developing cardiovascular disease. Those who averaged eight or more servings a day were 30 percent less likely to have had a heart attack or stroke than those eating less. Leafy green vegetables such as lettuce, spinach, Swiss chard, mustard greens; cruciferous vegetables such as broccoli, cauliflower, cabbage, Brussels sprouts, bok choy, and kale; and citrus fruit such as oranges, lemons, limes, and grapefruit seem to have the greatest benefit.

## Cancer

Scientists have long noted that there is a strong link between eating plenty of vegetables and fruit and protection against certain cancers. The International Agency for Research on Cancer, which is part of the World Health Organization, conducted a huge review of the best research on fruit, vegetables, and cancer. The study concluded that consumption of fruit and vegetables helped prevent cancers of the mouth and pharynx, esophagus, stomach, colon-rectum, larynx, lung, ovary, bladder, and kidney. They noted that eating more vegetables lowers the risk of cancers of the esophagus and colon-rectum and may reduce the risk of cancers of the mouth, pharynx, stomach, larynx, lung, ovaries, and kidneys.

### High Blood Pressure

A study called the DASH (the Dietary Approaches to Stop Hypertension) found that a diet rich in fruit, vegetables, and low-fat dairy products was able to significantly reduce the blood pressure of the subjects by as much as if they had used blood pressure–lowering medications. Because high blood pressure is a risk factor for heart disease and stroke, this is a significant finding.

### High Cholesterol

The National Heart, Lung, and Blood Institute's Family Heart Study found that eating more vegetables and fruit helps lower cholesterol. This large study followed more than four thousand men and women who ate at least three servings of vegetables and fruit a day. Those with the highest daily consumption (more than four servings a day) had significantly lower levels of LDL (bad cholesterol) than those with lower consumption. The researchers speculated that the participants' higher intake of vegetables and fruit limited how much meat and dairy they were consuming. Another possibility is that the fiber in vegetables and fruit actually blocks the absorption of cholesterol from food.

### Vision Problems

The Age-Related Eye Disease Study (AREDS) showed that a daily supplement of 500 milligrams of vitamin C, 400 international units of vitamin E, 15 milligrams of beta-carotene (often as vitamin A—up to 25,000 international units), 80 milligrams of zinc (as zinc oxide), and

*(Continued)*

2 milligrams of copper (as cupric oxide) reduced the risk of progressing to moderate or severe vision loss by up to 25 percent. Consuming vegetables and fruit, either juiced or whole, provides a host of these nutrients and reduces the chances of developing cataracts or macular degeneration. The provitamin A in carrots (known as carotenes), a favorite for juicing, promotes good vision. The phytonutrients in blueberries help improve night vision. And leafy dark-green vegetables are especially helpful because they contain two pigments, lutein and zeaxanthin, which attack free radicals before they can damage the eyes. There are many other vegetables and fruits that help prevent these two common eye diseases, which are frequently seen in Americans over the age of sixty-five.

Fresh juice not only contains most of the nutrients found in whole vegetables and fruit; it is also easily digested, thus providing good nutrient absorption. In addition, fresh vegetable juices are very alkalizing, so they are extremely beneficial to assist the body in detoxifying, which enables us to further resist disease, lose weight, and heal our bodies.

I have lectured and taught extensively about juicing. I've heard hundreds of personal testimonies from people who have been healed from numerous ailments ranging from heart disease to arthritis, chronic fatigue syndrome, fibromyalgia, and cancer. I know that incorporating fresh vegetable juices into your diet will assist your body in losing weight, healing, and rejuvenating. The nutrients in fresh juice help repair damaged cells and keep healthy cells strong. Once you remove as many of the sources of toxicity as possible by changing your diet to healthy choices, add fresh vegetable juice, and follow the cleansing programs outlined in the pages that follow, your body can remove irritating substances and restore healthy balance.

**Margo's Story**

I started juicing because I wanted better health and because I had lots of digestive problems. I had no idea that I'd also get rid of the pain in my left foot, and I could hardly walk before. I've noticed that my eyes are brighter, too.

## What About the Fiber?

Fiber is the portion of the plant that moves food through the digestive system. It is generally categorized as either soluble or insoluble. Both types of fiber help increase bulk, soften stools, and shorten the transit time of food moving through the intestinal tract. Both soluble and insoluble fibers are present in whole plant foods like vegetables, fruit, legumes, and grains. There is only soluble fiber in juice.

Soluble fiber in the form of pectins, gums, and mucilages partially dissolves in water, forming a type of gel; it is not digested. Soluble fiber absorbs digestive bile, which is made from cholesterol. When it's eliminated, it causes more cholesterol to be converted to digestive bile, thereby lowering LDL cholesterol. Soluble fiber also helps sugar to be more slowly absorbed, which helps regulate blood sugar and control diabetes. The best vegetable sources of soluble fiber are broccoli, carrots, Brussels sprouts, sweet potatoes, turnips, beets, squash, and pumpkin, all of which can be juiced. Soluble fiber is also found in nuts, legumes, barley, flaxseeds, psyllium husks, and oats and oat bran.

Insoluble fiber is also indigestible, but it does not dissolve in water. It absorbs water and serves as a bulking agent as it passes through the digestive system. Insoluble fiber promotes regular bowel movements and prevents constipation, as well as helps maintain a balanced pH in the intestines. It is important in cleansing because it removes toxic substances that tend to accumulate in the colon. Insoluble fiber is abundant in vegetables like leafy dark-green vegetables, green beans, and root vegetable skins, along with fruit skins and whole grains like oats, corn bran, seeds, and nuts.

In the past it was thought that a significant amount of nutrients remained in the fiber of fruits and vegetables after juicing, but that theory has been disproved. The Department of Agriculture analyzed twelve fruits in 1996 and found that 90 percent of the antioxidant activity was in the juice rather than the fiber.

It was also thought that juice had no fiber. Juicing got a bad rap in the early nineties that lingers on to this day. The media focused on the lack of fiber in juice. But that assertion was simply not true; the insoluble fiber is removed in the juicing process but some of the soluble fiber remains, which is excellent for the intestinal tract. A new study has disproved the idea that even the removal of the insoluble fiber makes fresh juice inferior. A 2006 review of eleven studies conducted by British researchers challenged the belief that fresh juices are not as beneficial as whole vegetables and fruit because they contain less fiber. The study, published in the *International Journal of Food Sciences and Nutrition,* found that "cancer and cardiovascular benefits may be more attributable to antioxidants rather than fibre." The researchers concluded that "[the theory that] pure fruit and vegetable juices are nutritionally inferior to [whole] fruit and vegetables, in relation to chronic disease risk reduction, is not justified."

The recommended fiber intake for adults is between 20 and 35 grams per day, but the average American's daily intake of dietary fiber is only around 14 to 15 grams. Increasing vegetable consumption by juicing will add to the daily intake of soluble fiber. In addition to fresh juice, eat more whole vegetables and fruit, include a leafy green salad every day, and eat plenty of nuts, seeds, legumes, and vegetables as part of a well-balanced, high-fiber diet. Adding flax fiber, psyllium husks, or other high-fiber bulking agents to your juice is another great way to increase your total fiber intake.

## THE COMPONENTS OF JUICE

In addition to fiber, fresh juice contains a wide variety of the nutrients that we need for health and wellness. The following list gives you a quick overview of what you get by adding fresh juice to your diet.

**Water.** Juice made from fresh produce provides an abundance of water, which is the body's most important nutrient. Water makes up 70 to 75 percent of total body weight and is involved in every bodily function. Water helps maintain body temperature, metabolizes body fat, generates energy, transports nutrients, and flushes toxins out of the body. It also lubricates joints and cushions delicate tissues and organs. Without adequate water, our bodies cannot function properly. Adding juice to your diet provides one of the most important requirements for health—water.

**Protein.** Also found in juice are a variety of amino acids, which are the building blocks of protein. Next to water, protein is the most plentiful component of our bodies. Protein is contained in every cell. It's needed to form structures like hair, skin, eyes, nails, muscles, connective tissue, and organs. It's also required for a host of biochemical processes. The body uses amino acids to build enzymes, which regulate chemical reactions and hormones.

Although vegetables and fruit contain incomplete protein, the amino acids are easily absorbed. Adding other protein sources, such as beans, lentils, dried peas, whole grains, and some free-range animal proteins, to your diet will supplement the vegetable protein in juice. Animal products like meat, poultry, fish, eggs, and dairy products contain the most complete form of protein. For some people, animal protein can be difficult to digest, and so more vegetable sources, such as legumes (beans, lentils, split peas), nuts, seeds, and whole grains, are required. Also, keep in mind that large quantities of animal protein can cause acidic by-products.

**Carbohydrates.** Juice contains an abundance of carbohydrates, which are the energy-producing substances that fuel our bodies. They are made up of simple sugar molecules, which are composed of the elements carbon, hydrogen, and oxygen. Complex carbohydrates, or starches, are basically chains of sugar molecules, often containing hundreds of these molecules. Carbohydrates are formed in plants when

they receive energy from the sun and store it in their chemical bonds. The energy contained in these carbohydrate molecules is released when the body metabolizes the plant food as
fuel. The three categories of carbohydrates are simple sugars,
complex carbohydrates, and fiber. Because fruit juice has a
high concentration of simple sugars, mainly fructose, it is recommended that you use fruit juice sparingly—no more than
4 ounces per day. On the other hand, you can drink large
amounts of vegetable juice. Vegetables and fruit contain both
soluble and insoluble fiber; juice contains only soluble fiber.

**Essential Fatty Acids (EFAs).** Juice contains only a small
amount of fatty acids. Because we need essential fats for
energy production and the formation of nerve cells, cellular
membranes, and special hormones like prostaglandins, we
need to supplement our diet with EFAs. A great way is to first
make some fresh juice with an emphasis on greens. Then
pour it into your blender and add an avocado, some ground
flaxseeds (a good source of omega-3 fatty acids), and blend;
this makes a satisfying and nourishing green smoothie.
You'll also need to supplement your diet with fish oil, krill
oil, cod liver oil, or flax oil for ample omega-3 fatty acids. And
you could include some omega-3–rich cold-water fish such
as wild-caught salmon (avoid farm raised). Your hair, skin,
joints, and heart will be happy!

**Vitamins.** Fresh juice is sometimes called "liquid vitamins" because it supplies so many of these vital nutrients. Vitamins are the organic nutrients required in small
amounts to maintain growth and normal metabolism. Most

vitamins serve as coenzymes and are part of many reactions in the body. The majority of vitamins can't be synthesized; they must be ingested. Fresh vegetable and fruit juices are excellent sources of water-soluble vitamins, principally many of the B complex vitamins (except B12, which is found in animal products), vitamin C, and phytochemicals. Fresh juice also contains some of the fat-soluble vitamins, notably carotenes (known as provitamin A), vitamin E, and vitamin K.

**Minerals.** A wide array of minerals is found in fresh juice. The major minerals in our bodies are calcium, chloride, magnesium, phosphorus, potassium, sodium, and sulfur. Trace minerals, which are required in very small amounts, include boron, chromium, cobalt, copper, fluoride, manganese, molybdenum, nickel, selenium, vanadium, and zinc. Our bodies need minerals for many functions such as bone and blood formation and to maintain the proper functioning of the cells. Along with vitamins, minerals are required for enzymes to function, particularly in the production of energy. Minerals are inorganic elements that plants absorb from the soil and then incorporate into their tissues by combining with organic molecules. These organic plant molecules can then be ingested in a highly usable form of juice that will provide us with the minerals we need to be healthy.

**Enzymes.** Biochemical processes can't take place in the body without the presence of enzymes. They are necessary for thousands of processes, such as metabolism, energy production, and the building and repair of cells. Enzymes have been called the "workforce" of the body, and without them, our cells would not survive. Fresh juice is loaded with enzymes because it's made from raw, live produce. Heating, as happens in cooking, blanching, pasteurization, or canning, destroys them. When we drink juice made from fresh vegetables and fruit we are supplying our bodies with an abundance of the enzymes needed to digest the food, which spares our organs from working overtime to supply enzymes. This allows the body's energy to be shifted from digestion to other functions such as repair and detoxification, which is one reason why people who regularly drink fresh juice usually notice that their energy levels increase.

**Biophotons.** Photons are light rays of energy that are found in the living cells of raw foods such as fruits and vegetables. They are a new frontier of research and have been shown to emit coherent light energy when uniquely photographed with a process known as Kirlian photography. This light energy is believed to have many benefits when consumed. Biophotons are believed to aid cellular communication and to feed the mitochondria, which produces ATP—our energy fuel, and the DNA. They are believed to contribute to our energy, vitality, and a feeling of vibrancy and well-being. They are easily destroyed by heat and processing.

**Phytochemicals.** Known as "plant chemicals," phytochemicals, also called phytonutrients, are produced by plants to protect them from disease, injury, and pollution. They also give plants their color, odor, and flavor. There are tens of thousands of phytochemicals in the vegetables and fruit we eat. For example, the average tomato may contain up to ten thousand different types of these nutrients. Phytochemicals are more resistant to heat than vitamins and enzymes, so they can withstand cooking. Nevertheless, drinking them in fresh juice provides much more concentration because we usually juice more than we could chew at one time.

Though they may sound like ingredients found in shampoo, phytochemicals such as allyl sulfides, curcumins, ellagic acid, gingerol, indoles, isothiocyanates, sulforaphanes, limonene, lycopene, and monoterpenes can prevent a host of diseases. Research shows that people who eat plenty of vegetables and fruit have the lowest incidence of cancer, particularly stomach, breast, lung, prostate, skin, liver, and pancreatic. They've also been shown to help reduce inflammation, lower cholesterol levels, fight viruses, heal ulcers, increase immune function, stimulate detoxification enzymes, and protect DNA from damage. Foods like garlic, onions, ginger, turmeric, strawberries, cruciferous vegetables (broccoli, cabbage, and cauliflower), citrus fruit, tomatoes, berries, and cherries are particularly rich in phytonutrients.

## Choosing the Best Juicer

Now that you know a lot about why juicing is good for you, all you need is a good juicer to get started. A juicer and a blender are different. A juicer separates the liquid juice from the pulp. You drink the juice and toss the pulp or compost it. On the other hand, a blender doesn't separate the pulp from the juice. Even the high-speed types simply whirl everything around and mix it up. You generally have to add some liquid like water or juice to get things going. Blenders are great for making smoothies and cold soups with soft produce, but they won't make juice. Blended hard vegetables such as carrots, beets, and stringy veggies like celery turn out quite mushy or gritty. If you try to make carrot juice with water and carrots in your blender, you'll have a very fiber-thick, mushy substance. I recommend you use a juicer for vegetable juice and a blender for smoothies and raw soups.

## FEATURES OF A GOOD JUICER

Choosing the right juicer will determine whether you become dedicated to juicing or try it a few times and never juice again. You can spend lots of money on some juicers, and though they may be good quality, many are a hassle to clean. You may save money on a chain store bargain, but it won't do you much good if it sits in your bottom cupboard because it's a big hassle to use or it doesn't juice well. Here's what to look for:

**Has Adequate Horsepower.** Choose a juicer that is at least one-third to one horsepower. Weak machines with low horsepower ratings must run at extremely high rpm (revolutions per minute). A machine's rpm does not accurately reflect its ability to perform effectively, because rpm is calculated when the juicer is running idle, not while it is juicing. However, when you feed produce into a low-power machine, the rpm will be reduced dramatically, and sometimes the juicer will come to a full stop. I have "killed" some machines on the first carrot I juiced.

**Maintains Blade Speed.** Look for a machine that has electronic circuitry that sustains blade speed during juicing.

**Doesn't Need Special Tool to Loosen Juicer Blade.** There are a few popular machines that require a special tool to get the blade out for washing and to tighten it again. Lose the tool and you can't use your juicer.

**Is Strong Enough for Hard Vegetables.** Make sure the machine can juice tough, hard vegetables, such as carrots and beets, as well as delicate greens, such as parsley, lettuce, and herbs.

**Doesn't Need Special Citrus Attachment.** Make sure you can use the juicer for citrus fruit such as lemons and limes.

**Has Large Feeding Tube.** This feature allows you to put whole or large pieces of produce in the juicer, so you don't have to cut everything up into little pieces, which saves significant time and energy.

**Ejects Pulp into Receptacle.** Choose a juicer that ejects the pulp into a receptacle. This design is far better than one in which all the pulp stays inside the machine and so has to be scooped out frequently. Juicers that keep the pulp in the center basket rather than ejecting it cannot juice continuously. You'll need to stop the machine often to wash it out. One time-saver—you can line the receptacle with a baggie, which eliminates the need for washing. That's one less part to hassle with.

**Has Few Parts to Clean.** Look for a juicer with only a

few parts to clean. The more parts a juicer has, and the more complicated the parts are to wash, the longer it will take to clean your juicer and put it back together. The fewer parts to clean, the more likely you'll be to use it daily. Also, make sure the parts are dishwasher safe.

Now it's time to begin juicing. I have plenty of delicious recipes for you in chapter ten and suggestions along the way. So grab your juicer, or go buy one, and get started juicing right away!

## Juicing Made Simple

Now that you know all about the best juicers, it's time to begin! If you're a little intimidated or puzzled about how to start, rest assured; it's really quite simple. Just follow these few easy steps and you're on your way.

STEP 1: **Buy enough produce to make the juice you want.** Figure out how much juice you want to make. I recommend at least one to two 8-ounce glasses a day per person, but you'll need more if you're cleansing or doing a juice fast. To make one 8-ounce glass of juice, you'll need about a pound of produce; for example, two or three carrots, half a lemon, one or two ribs of celery, and a cucumber. You may want to add leafy green vegetables like spinach, kale, or parsley, which can be strong tasting, so it's always best to mix them with mild-tasting vegetables.

**STEP 2: Wash all the produce before juicing.** Washing your produce is something you can do ahead of time. Store it in the refrigerator in glass or plastic containers or green produce bags so it's ready to juice later. Most health food stores and many grocery stores have vegetable washes that you can purchase for removing toxins and dirt. (Be aware that washes cannot remove pesticides that are systemic, meaning that they are found throughout the plant.) Or you can fill your sink or a large container with sea salt and wash the produce in the salt solution. Use a vegetable brush to remove the dirt, even for organic produce.

**STEP 3: Prepare the produce.** Be sure to cut off any parts that are bruised, moldy, or damaged. Peel the following:

- Anything not labeled organic should be peeled, as the pesticides are concentrated in the peel (unfortunately, so are the nutrients).
- Always peel oranges, grapefruits, tangerines, and tangelos, as they contain volatile oils that can make you sick.
- Lemons and limes don't have to be peeled if they are organic, but many people like to peel them since the skin can be a little bitter or strong tasting.

What to take out and what to leave in:

- **Take out** pits, stones, and hard seeds.
- **Leave in** softer seeds such as pear and apple seeds.

- **Leave on** the stems and leaves of most produce, such as beet greens and parsley stems, as there's a lot of nutritional value in them; take off hard stems.
- **Cut off** carrot greens because they contain toxic substances.

**STEP 4: Start cutting things up.** Cut the vegetables and fruit (primarily lemon, lime, or green apple) into sections that will fit your juicer's feed tube. Many of the new juicers have very wide feeding tubes that enable you to put in whole small beets, tomatoes, small apples, small lemons, limes, and large carrots, without cutting them at all. Larger items like cabbage, cauliflower, and so forth obviously need to be cut into smaller pieces. It won't take you long to figure out what works with your juicer.

**STEP 5: Prepare to catch the pulp.** Line the pulp receptacle with a plastic bag; you can use the free ones you get in the grocery store produce section. When you're finished juicing, toss the baggie with the pulp or throw it in your compost pile. Then you won't have to wash out the receptacle—saving you even more time.

**STEP 6: Prepare to catch the juice.** This may seem obvious, but unless your juicer comes with its own container to catch the juice (some do; most don't), you'll need to find a container that is tall enough and wide enough so the juice doesn't end up on the counter. You could use a 4-cup glass

Pyrex measuring cup, but any container will do, as long as it's the right size.

**STEP 7: What to do with produce you can't juice.** Avocados don't juice well since they don't contain enough water. Add them to juices like carrot, lemon, and cucumber by combining them in a blender. This makes a delicious satisfying cold soup or smoothie. Bananas won't juice either, but they work well in a smoothie.

**STEP 8: Drink your juice!** If possible, it's best to drink your juice as soon as it's prepared. Freshly made juice contains the most nutrients; the longer it sits, the more it loses. If you need to make juice ahead of time because you can't juice in the morning or during the day, then store it in an insulated container like a thermos, or another type of airtight, opaque container in the refrigerator. You can store it for up to twenty-four hours. It will still lose some nutrients, but it's far better than anything you can buy already bottled. Many of the nutrients like vitamins, enzymes, biophotons, and some phytochemicals are affected by light and heat, which causes them to oxidize or destroys them. As you might guess, if the juice turns brown, that's a sign that it has oxidized and has lost a good share of its nutritional value. Cabbage juice should be consumed as soon as you make it, as it does not store well.

*On a personal note:* When I had chronic fatigue syndrome, I would juice in the afternoons, when I had the most energy, and store the juice covered in the refrigerator and drink it for the next twenty-four hours until I juiced my next batch. I got well doing this, so I can assure you that a lot of nutrients remained intact even though refrigerated for up to twenty-four hours.

## Choose Organic Produce

The best way to get the healthiest juice possible is to buy organic produce whenever you can. It is even more important when you're on a cleansing program to avoid ingesting pesticides and other toxic products—the very stuff you're trying to get rid of. Certified organic vegetables and fruit are grown without pesticides, fungicides, herbicides, or chemical fertilizers. And organic farmers don't use genetically modified seeds. Always look for food that is labeled "certified organic." This means the produce has been cultivated according to strict uniform standards that are verified by independent state or private organizations. Certification includes inspection of farms and processing facilities, detailed record keeping, and pesticide testing of soil and water to ensure that growers and handlers are meeting government standards.

Researchers say there is now firm evidence that choosing organic foods helps you avoid toxic pesticides. In 1995 the USDA tested nearly seven thousand conventionally grown fruit and vegetable samples and detected residues of sixty-five different pesticides, with two out of three samples containing pesticide residue.

In recent years, increased awareness among the health-conscious public has made organic foods much easier to find. Many grocery stores now have organic sections and health food stores and natural foods chains have sprung up across the country. There are organic food co-ops, buying clubs, and organic farmers' markets in nearly every part of the country. The sale of organic foods has become a multibillion-dollar industry. As more people become educated about the wholesale use of pesticides and herbicides and the negative health effects, they are demanding organic food. That's because pesticide residues have been shown to cause numerous long-term health risks, such as cancer and birth defects, and immediate health risks from acute intoxication, such as vomiting, diarrhea, blurred vision, tremors, convulsions, and nerve damage.

Many studies have shown that organically grown vegetables and fruit have been found to have higher concentrations of vitamins and minerals than those that are cultivated inorganically. While organic foods are always the best option in terms of avoiding pesticides, studies also show they are higher in nutrient content. In a 2001 study published in the *Journal of Alternative and Complementary Medicine*, on average, organic produce contained 27 percent more vitamin C, 21 percent more iron, and 29 percent more magnesium than conventional produce, and all twenty-one minerals compared in the study were higher in the organic produce. Additionally, research has shown that organic food contains more secondary metabolites than conventionally grown plants. Secondary metabolites are substances that form part of the plants' immune system, and that helps fight cancer in humans.

Chemical fertilizers can reduce the quality of nutrition. For example, the quality of protein in grains and vegetables is related to the amount of nitrogen in the soil. When there is a lot of nitrogen present, plants increase protein production and decrease carbohydrate synthesis. When the metabolic protein requirements are satisfied, the remaining protein produced is stored in a form that contains fewer essential amino acids. The result of high levels of nitrogen, as found in conventional chemical fertilizers, is an increase in the amount of protein but a reduction in its quality. Organically managed soils release nitrogen in smaller amounts over a longer time than conventional fertilizers. As a result, the quality of protein from organic crops is better in terms of human nutrition.

If you'd like to stay informed about the latest information on organic foods and have a political voice regarding our food, go to OrganicConsumers.org and sign up for the free e-newsletter. It's interesting and informative and gives you opportunities to make your voice heard politically.

In addition to choosing organically grown food, check carefully to see if the vegetables and fruit have been irradiated. The FDA requires that irradiated foods include labeling with either the statement "treated with radiation" or "treated by irradiation," along with the international symbol for irradiation, the Radura. Irradiation labeling requirements apply only to foods sold in stores. For example, irradiated spices or fresh strawberries should be labeled. But irradiation labeling is not required for restaurant foods. Irradiation, known as gamma-ray radiation, is used to kill pests and germs in stored food, which seems to improve the shelf life of the food, but it doesn't preserve your life. Even though the FDA allows its use, radiation doses for food decontamination can be up to five million times that of a typical chest X-ray. They may kill the bugs, but they also generate free radicals in the food that, when ingested, can damage your cells. In addition, the practice destroys vitamins and minerals.

### Avoid the "Dirty Dozen"

The nonprofit research organization Environmental Working Group reports periodically on health risks posed by pesticides in produce. The group says you can cut your pesticide exposure by almost 90 percent by avoiding the top twelve conventionally grown vegetables and fruit that are the most contaminated; purchase only organic for these twelve. Using this guide will help you make wise choices. Each year the list changes a bit. You can always go to EWG.org and check out the most up-to-date rankings for the year. Whenever you are on a cleansing program, it is vitally important to consume food that is as pesticide-free as possible.

**THE DIRTY DOZEN LIST**

(From EWG.org, as of May 2012, ranked in order, with the worst at number 1.)

1. Apples
2. Celery
3. Strawberries
4. Peaches
5. Spinach
6. Nectarines
7. Grapes (This covers raisins and wine, too.)
8. Sweet Bell Peppers
9. Potatoes
10. Blueberries
11. Lettuce
12. Kale/Collard Greens

You don't have to choose everything from the organic section. The Clean Fifteen lists the produce with the least pesticides. Each year, the Environmental Working Group publishes the list of the least offenders; see EWG.org.

**THE CLEAN FIFTEEN FOOD LIST**

(From EWG.org, as of May 2012, ranked in order, with the best at number 1.)

1. Onions
2. Sweet Corn
3. Pineapples
4. Avocados
5. Asparagus
6. Sweet Peas
7. Mangoes
8. Eggplant
9. Cantaloupe (domestic)
10. Kiwi
11. Cabbage
12. Watermelon
13. Sweet Potatoes
14. Grapefruit
15. Mushrooms

**Note:** Since carrots are used often in juice recipes, be aware that they are usually ranked between number 13 and number 15 on the list of foods containing the highest amount of pesticides; therefore, it's important to buy organic carrots.

## Genetically Modified Foods

Whenever possible, avoid genetically modified foods, also known as GMs or GMOs. Scientists, doctors, and health educators in many sectors of the health industry have long warned about the possible deleterious effects of GM crops on the health of animals and humans. An Australian project to develop genetically modified peas with built-in pest resistance had to be abandoned after tests showed they caused allergic lung damage in mice. A similar situation occurred in the early 1990s when a strain of bioengineered soybeans was found to cause an allergic response in people with Brazil nut allergies.

A March 2007 article in the journal *Archives of Environmental Contamination and Toxicology* reported on a study that was commissioned by the environmental group Greenpeace in which rats were fed for ninety days on GM maize (corn) developed by the chemical giant Monsanto. The rats showed signs of toxicity in the liver and kidneys. In reporting on this study, *Scientific American* quoted a statement by then Greenpeace spokesman Arnaud Apoteker: "It is the first time that independent research, published in a peer-reviewed journal, has proved that a GMO authorized for human consumption presents signs of toxicity."

A genetically modified organism (GMO) is an organism whose genetic material has been altered using bioengineering techniques. GMO foods have raised concerns because they force genetic information across the protective species barrier in an unnatural way. In other words, nature does not sustain them. These new organisms are in many cases untested, yet they are on grocery store shelves everywhere without protective labeling. We may not know we are buying them.

The United States is the main supplier of GMO seeds worldwide, and the crops are virtually uncontrolled in this country. President Obama signed the "Monsanto Protection Act" into law in March 2013. It grants Monsanto and the entire biotech industry the power to nullify federal courts, even when those courts determine that particular GMO crops may be dangerous to human health or the environment. On the other hand, many countries around the world have banned their use, including many in the European Union that are fighting to keep their crops pure. Hungary, one of Europe's biggest grain producers, became the first country in Eastern Europe to ban GMO crops or foods when it outlawed the planting of maize seeds marketed by Monsanto, in January 2005. As it stands now, we have about a 70 to 75 percent chance of picking a product with GMO ingredients without even realizing it. This is astounding! We need to take notice when we're selecting food to support our health, particularly if we are cleansing to remove toxins. We can make our voices heard that we don't want GMO crops grown in the United States by not purchasing the top GMO foods including soy and corn. We can also vote for GMO labeling.

The small stickers attached to fresh produce can tell you more about the food than you think.

The four- to five-digit codes, called price lookup codes (PLUs), are used worldwide to enable stores to track inventory and scan prices at checkout. These labels can also help us determine where the food came from. We can even identify genetically modified food. The labels also help us spot the difference between fruits like Fuji and Gala apples. All produce, including fruits, vegetables, dried fruit, herbs, and nuts, gets a label.

Here's your guide to reading the labels:

- **Conventionally grown fruit:** Produce bearing these four-digit numbers runs the gamut from guava to kiwi. For example, guava is 4299 and a banana is 4011. You can also search PLU codes online.
- **Organically grown fruit:** This produce has five-digit labels that start with the number 9. An organically grown banana would be 94011.

*(Continued)*

- **Genetically modified food:** These five-digit labels start with an 8, so a genetically engineered vine-ripened tomato would be 84805.

  You can read more at the BusinessInsider.com article "Here's What the Sticker on Your Produce Really Means."

We can avoid GMO foods by becoming aware of which foods are most prone to genetic engineering and what products are made from them. To date, the biggest GM crops are soybeans and corn, from which thousands of processed foods are made. Look at the labels on all products you purchase to see if they contain corn flour or cornmeal, soy flour, cornstarch, textured vegetable protein, corn syrup, or modified food starch. Check labels of soy sauce, tofu, soy beverages, soy protein isolate, soy milk, soy ice cream, margarine, soy lecithin, among dozens of other products. If the label doesn't say organic, the chances are strong that it's GMO. It's particularly important to choose organic soy or corn products to ensure that they are not GMO. Aside from corn and soy, other GMO foods grown in the United States include cotton (cottonseed oil), canola, sugar beets, squash, and papaya. You can vote with your dollars by purchasing only products labeled organic, especially when it comes to foods and by-products of food that are likely to be grown from GMO crops.

Become an informed consumer. The FDA has refused to require labeling of genetically engineered foods, despite overwhelming American support for mandatory labeling. Since the agency has refused to protect consumers, some food companies are now taking action by labeling certain prod-ucts or ingredients "non-GMO," which means "made with-out genetically modified organisms." The United States may soon be the only country in the world that does not require labeling of genetically engineered food.

### Juicing for Life: Summary

**Step 1:** Continue eating whole foods and alkalizing foods, using organic, non-GMO products, removing as many sources of toxicity as possible, drinking plenty of water, and eating at least 50 percent raw foods.

**Step 2:** Add fresh vegetable juices to your diet at least once or twice a day.

# CHAPTER THREE

## Juice Fasting for Life

Juice fasting, or juice feasting as it's become known, is an excellent way to lose weight and cleanse the body of toxins, but it is much more than that. Its virtues have been extolled for centuries by nearly every religious practice as a way to connect to something higher and more significant than oneself and the needs of one's body. Fasting can make you feel lighter, happier, healthier, and more focused. The air will seem clearer, colors brighter, and sights and sounds sharper and more beautiful.

Fasting literally means to abstain from all or certain types of food and drink. It can mean a lot of different things, such as fasting from sugar, alcohol, coffee, meat, dairy, or whatever else one chooses to give up. There are many types of fasts and methods of fasting. Some of these methods are quite controversial. For instance, one type of fasting, known as total fasting, is to take nothing in by mouth—not food or water. I consider a total fast dangerous. Our bodies need 2 to 2 1/2 quarts of water a day to function well. Without adequate water, dehydration can occur, electrolyte balance is disturbed, and the delicate tissues of the body can become damaged.

Another type is the water-only fast. This fast involves totally abstaining from all solid or liquid food and drinking only water. I don't recommend water-only fasting unless you've completed a number of cleansing programs and some vegetable-juice fasting beforehand and are working with a health professional to supervise this fast, because fasting causes toxins to be rapidly released into the bloodstream. Without an ample supply of antioxidants from your diet, provided with vegetable juices, the large amount of toxins released with fasting could damage your cells. Antioxidants bind to toxins and carry them out of the body so they don't cause damage. I use vegetable-juice fasting because vegetable juices are loaded with antioxidants and are very alkalizing. This is a safe and effective way to cleanse your body's internal organs, tissues, and cells. Vegetable-juice fasting supports detoxification by providing nutrients, with an abundance of antioxidants like vitamins C and E, beta-carotene, selenium, and various enzymes and phytochemicals that bind to and neutralize toxins.

When you fast, you are voluntarily setting aside the

temptations of food, the ritual of eating, and the demands of your cravings. In exchange for the discipline of forgoing solid food for a period of time, you'll have a chance to reflect on the deeper aspects of your soul, such as your purpose and what is truly important in life. Fasting can free you from addictions and dependencies of all kinds. It can give you the sense of control over your body that allows you to consider new ways of living and new possibilities. You'll see creative solutions to problems more clearly when you are not weighed down with the burden of food preparation and digestion. And your body and soul are given a chance to heal.

During Lent, the monks at some monasteries chant, "Through abstinence, what is tired and weak and sick becomes strong." This is actually true. You'll become stronger because of your fast. This might seem like a contradiction, since we think of food as a key to strength. Indeed, healthy food does make you strong. But there is a place for abstinence from food as well in the rhythm of life, and fasting will also strengthen and renew your body and soul.

Fasting is energizing because you are resting your body from the work of digestion. Normally, about 30 percent of our overall energy expenditure is devoted to digestion. Think of it—you'll have 30 percent more energy freed up just by not eating!

When you fast, this energy can be used for healing, repair, and restoration of your body. Without solid food being ingested throughout the day, the body looks for new sources of fuel to burn for energy. It first draws on readily available glucose that is stored in the liver as glycogen. Next it turns to other sources like the fatty acids in fat cells and proteins that are most readily available. Then it turns to sick or damaged cells. The body is continually making new cells and breaking down old, sick, or damaged ones. Of the trillions of cells in our bodies, it is estimated that about one-fourth, or around three to eight hundred billion, are broken down and replaced daily. During fasting, the process of degrading sick cells is accelerated. Their raw materials are then recycled to be used either as energy or as building blocks for new cells. Those that cannot be used are eliminated. This explains why skin starts to look so much younger and more vibrant during a fast and why the body starts getting well.

When you fast for a few days, many cravings go away and thoughts about food usually diminish. You have time to focus on other things. This gives your body a chance to use its energy for clearing out old waste that has accumulated in both your body and your mind. Many people report a spiritual experience during this time. Other people are simply joyful because they feel in control of their appetite for the first time in years or are making progress on health improvement or weight management. Others, though, notice that they are more irritable or angry. Emotions are often released when we fast.

Just like many things that are good for us, fasting has gotten a bad rap in our culture. We're so inundated with advertising that tells us we have to constantly consume food that the very idea of going without it—on purpose—is contrary to everything we're conditioned to believe.

You may be thinking that fasting is something so difficult that you can't possibly do it, or that it's only for those super-disciplined people who don't suffer from any of the challenges you've had when you tried fasting in the past. I understand, because I've been there. However, I can promise you that fasting doesn't have to involve unnecessary pain or discomfort. Let me encourage you to give it a try. Millions of people throughout time have fasted successfully. And, thankfully, you don't have to white-knuckle it through a difficult water fast. A short vegetable-juice fast is something that almost anyone can do, including you. You can happily fast for a day or two with fresh juices, smoothies, and cold soups and feel good in the process. Later, if you choose, you can go on a longer fast and enjoy even greater benefits.

Since fasting involves abstaining from food, many people have a negative reaction when they think about it. Some people focus on denial and the possibility of discomfort. Some are fearful of weakness or detox symptoms, but most of the symptoms are due to the release of toxins that have accumulated through the years; these toxins are what will make our bodies sick in the long run. Release of toxins is exactly what we want our bodies to do. So don't worry. I'll show you how to prepare for a fast so detox symptoms should be minor and pass quickly. I'll help you through your fast with tips to make it easier, and I'll show you how to successfully break a fast. And the rewards you'll get will be great.

### Michele's Story

I never wanted to try fasting because I believed it would make me feel weak and sick. Because I was diagnosed with hypoglycemia (low blood sugar), I believed that I had to eat something every few hours, especially protein. My only experience with fasting was when I would try to do some sort of cleansing routine for my colon or liver, which was usually very unpleasant because I did it incorrectly.

When I began to learn about all the wonderful benefits of fasting, I decided to try it. First I did a one-day juice fast that included fresh vegetable juices and some smoothies made with vegetable juice and avocados. I felt so good I decided to try it for another two days. After three days of vegetable-juice fasting I felt full of energy and very clearheaded. And I was grateful to be freed from the chore of having to think about what I had to prepare to eat and what not to eat each day. I lost several pounds, too, although this was not my reason for the fast. I was amazed at how good I felt and decided to try it again the next week. Although I had a few detox symptoms, like a headache and a little weakness periodically, most of the time I felt incredibly well and was able to do moderate exercises. After completing the fast, I increased the intensity and time of my workouts in the gym. I literally felt like running a marathon on some of the days. I also noticed greater mental clarity and spiritual focus.

For me it was important to lead up to my fast with proper preparation. Cherie recommended that I add daily vegetable juicing to my diet for about two weeks before the fast, plus I ate almost 80 percent of my food fresh and raw. I believe the preparation enabled me to get through the fast with minimal discomfort.

I've noticed that many of the symptoms that have plagued me for years are mostly gone, as long as I don't overeat. I no longer have digestive problems like constipation or acid reflux. My weight is normal and my energy is high. My skin is clear and bright and my mental clarity is great, even though I'm over fifty. I'm now a dedicated juice faster and I tell all my friends about it and encourage them to try it too.

## The Juice Feast Reboot

Have you seen the movie *Fat, Sick, and Nearly Dead*? It's the story of Joe Cross, who was 100 pounds overweight (he weighed 310 pounds) and had a gut bigger than a beach ball.

Loaded up on steroids, he suffered from a debilitating auto-immune disease called chronic urticaria. Chronic urticaria is a rare disorder that results in the constant outbreak of hives even when the individual is not exposed to an allergen or other normal triggers. It causes a great deal of pain and suffering. While chronic urticaria is managed by loads of medication, it cannot currently be cured by any known means available to Western medicine. For Joe Cross, the condition finally became too much to bear.

This inspiring film chronicles Joe's personal mission to regain his health. With doctors and conventional medicines unable to help him, Joe turned to the only option he had left, his body's ability to heal itself. He traded in the junk food for a juicer and a bunch of fruits and vegetables and hit the road with the juicer and a generator in tow, vowing to drink *only* fresh fruit and vegetable juice for the next sixty days. Across three thousand miles Joe has one goal in mind—to get off his pills, regain his health, and achieve a balanced lifestyle. While on his journey, he talks to more than five hundred Americans about food, health, and longevity, but it's at a truck stop in Arizona that he meets a truck driver who suffers from the same rare condition. Phil Staples was morbidly obese, weighing in at 429 pounds—a cheeseburger away from a heart attack. As Joe is regaining his health, Phil is inspired to begin his own epic journey to get well. What emerges is nothing short of amazing. During the sixty-day juice fast (or juice feast), Joe lost between 80 and 85 pounds. For three months after that, he stuck to plant foods and was down to 210 pounds—a 100-pound weight loss. Phil, the truck driver from Iowa, lost 180 pounds. And for both of them, their chronic urticaria stopped flaring up and they no longer needed their medications.

## Why Juice Fasting Helps Us Heal, Lose Weight, and Look Younger

Each of the trillions of cells in our bodies has a permeable membrane that enables it to take in nutrients and excrete waste. Cell membranes often become hardened, or rigid; thus, the cells cannot properly excrete toxins trapped within them. Much of the reason for cell wall rigidity is the acidity of toxic waste that is caused by eating too much acid-producing food, constant stress, negative thoughts and emotions, and environmental toxins. The acidity in the fluids surrounding the cells changes them and they become hardened.

When the cells are not properly able to excrete the buildup of toxic and acidic waste, this condition affects their ability to produce energy. This is because the mitochondria, little structures within the cells that generate ATP (a form of chemical energy), become much less efficient at their assigned task of producing energy. The result is that we feel tired, worn-out, and lethargic and we start looking older.

Along comes vegetable-juice fasting to the rescue. It alkalizes the cells and the surrounding fluids, which renews cells so they can dump waste, while supplying antioxidant nutrients that help neutralize the toxins. Fasting restores an alkaline pH balance and enables cell walls to return to their ideal, permeable state. Once the cell membranes are softened, the process of dumping wastes is accelerated. Now the cells can again function at peak efficiency, something they may not have been able to do for many years. Many people lose weight at that point.

Alkalizing and cleansing your body helps you lose weight. The body is very intelligent. As we become more and more acidic, it sets up defense mechanisms to keep the damaging acid from entering our vital organs. We know that acid gets stored in fat cells. After all, if the acid comes into contact with our organs, it can damage them and cause cells to mutate. Also, the oxygen level drops in an acidic environment, which sets up an environment for cancer cells to thrive. And calcium becomes depleted in an acidic environment, which is a setup for osteoporosis. So as a defense mechanism, your body may actually make fat to protect you from an overly acidic internal environment. Those fat cells and cellulite deposits (that lumpy, bumpy, orange-peel skin) may actually be packing up the acid to keep it at a safe distance from your organs. When your body starts dumping toxins, it can also let go of fat because it doesn't need it anymore. And, voilà! That stubborn, hard-to-lose pudge just seems to melt away—sometimes quite rapidly. This fat loss may not be due as much to reduction in calories as it is to flushing away acidic, toxic waste. This truly is an "eat and grow thin" possibility.

One more reason to juice fast is to give your organs

of digestion a rest. When we eat solid food, they must spend a lot of our waking hours digesting all that food. But when we juice fast, our nutrition comes in a predigested form that is easily used. That spares our digestive system hours of work. It can focus on healing and repair. Many people notice a great improvement in their health during or after a juice feast.

## The Physical Benefits of Juice Fasting

- Increases energy and strength
- Detoxifies cells and tissues
- Assists in weight loss
- Improves mental clarity
- Restores alkaline balance
- Strengthens the immune system
- Helps prevent disease
- Tightens skin
- Smoothes wrinkles
- Lowers blood pressure
- Lowers cholesterol
- Lessens aches and pains
- Revitalizes organ systems
- Rests the gastrointestinal system
- Balances the nervous system
- Increases ease of movement
- Helps the lungs breathe more deeply

## Preparing to Fast

If you decide to do a one-day juice fast, then just jump right in and go for it! It doesn't have to be difficult or complicated or take a lot of preparation. Almost anyone can do well on a one-day vegetable-juice fast and will feel better for it. If you've never fasted before, start with one day. Many people like to start on a Friday evening with veggie juice for dinner and then for breakfast and lunch the next day, and break the fast that evening with a big salad. Most people do best if they start out slowly and then add more fast days later on. But you might be like Joe Cross and Phil Staples—desperate for change.

The following suggestions for fasting will help you tremendously if you decide to do two, three, or more days of fasting. There are people who routinely do five- to ten-day juice fasts, which is where many of the most transforming benefits are realized. And some people, like Joe and Phil, juice feast for sixty days or more.

Listen to your body if you decide to fast for longer than three days. If you want to have a successful two- or three-day fast with all the benefits that have been described, it's best to prepare properly before you begin. I have found this to be a very important step for anyone who is beginning a fast. Should you decide to begin with a two- or three-day fast, it will help if you lead up to it. Follow the guidelines "Making Wise Food Choices" on page 33 in chapter one.

Additionally, one week before your fast, eat smaller portions than usual. Most of us can get by on about half of our usual serving sizes, so it's a great idea to practice eating only enough to satisfy your hunger. Also, eat more raw vegetables and fruit, making about 75 to 80 percent of your diet raw. This will slowly help detoxify and alkalize your body so you will have fewer detox symptoms when you fast.

Many people fail at fasting because they go straight into a water-only or juice fast without any preparation or transition. If you jump from the typical American diet into a several-day fast, you could feel quite sick and swear you'll never do that again. Lots of people do a pig-out before they start a fast; that's really not a good idea. Resist the temptation to have a big last supper before you fast. Ease into your fast and prepare for it.

Exercise is also important in any cleansing program. If you are not accustomed to regular exercise, begin now by walking, bicycling, slow jogging, rebounding, using the lymphasizer (see pages 209–11), or dancing. If you haven't had any exercise for a while, start with fifteen to thirty minutes and work up to more time. Make sure you do something that encourages a lot of deep breathing. And ease into it with something not too strenuous, like walking or rebounding. Competitive or intense workouts are not good starter exercises; you could end up so sore you won't be able to exercise for quite a while, or worse yet, you could tear a muscle. Also incorporate regular stretching exercises into your daily routine. And don't forget to take plenty of deep breaths throughout the day.

## CONSIDER YOUR MOTIVES FOR FASTING

Do you just want to lose weight, or are you fasting for improved health and wellness or for spiritual reasons? It helps to have a clear idea about your goals when you start. If you want to cleanse and purify your body so you can increase your energy, mental clarity, and spiritual growth, write these goals down to remind yourself later when you may have a weak moment.

Fasting requires discipline, commitment, and determination. If you're in the right frame of mind when you start, it will be much easier. There are always temptations to pull you away from your commitment. Your family and friends may offer you a tempting dish, telling you, "Just one bite won't hurt." That's why it helps to write down your reasons for fasting, or tell a friend who will support you or even join you. It also helps to get away for a while, for instance, to a retreat or a spa that offers juice fasting (see the Resources Guide for information on my juice fast and raw foods retreats). If this is not possible, then begin to clear your schedule. Say no to commitments for a few days. Turn off the radio, television, and computer. This is a time to rest, relax, go to bed early, and give your body a chance to restore and heal. Remind yourself that it's just for a little while. The world will actually go on functioning without you! If you have family or work commitments, try to minimize any extra involvement with the outside world.

Prepare yourself mentally and physically by reading, exercising, praying, or just being still. You might want to take a day of relaxation before you begin your fast so you can calm your body and mind and reflect on what you want to gain from your fast. You will be most successful if you seek peace and serenity while you fast.

## WHO SHOULD NOT FAST

Fasting is safe and beneficial for most people, yet some people should not fast, and others should fast only with supervision, including the following:

- People with diabetes, particularly those on insulin (choose option two on page 85)

- People with hypoglycemia (although many with blood sugar imbalances do well on a short vegetable-juice fast, especially if it's modified—see option two on page 85)

- Children under eighteen (unless recommended by a health professional)

- People with anemia, wasting as with advanced stages of cancer, or extreme weakness

- People with a very aggressive cancer; however, modified fasts may be appropriate (see option two on page 85).

- People with eating disorders such as anorexia or bulimia

- Women who are pregnant or nursing

- People with a serious health problem; these individuals may need professional supervision

- People with concerns about fasting; these individuals should consult a health professional

## How to Juice Fast

Now that you have decided to juice fast for one, two, three, or more days and you've set aside the time and cleared your schedule, you can relax and settle into the adventure of juice fasting. Take a look at the recipes you want to make. Now it's time to make your shopping list. Make sure you have on hand plenty of fresh organic vegetables and a few low-sugar fruits, such as lemons, limes, or green apples, so you don't have to run to the store on your fasting days.

You can drink as much vegetable juice as you like and as often as you like. Some people choose to make a variety of juices throughout the day; others prefer to make one big batch (several glasses to a quart or two) of juice at one time and sip it throughout the day. It's up to you. If you do make the juice ahead of time, keep it in an airtight container to preserve as many of the enzymes and vitamins as possible. Some people make a really large batch and freeze some of the juice in individual containers. Glass is what I recommend, but don't fill the jars to the top. The juice will expand when it freezes and break the jar, so leave a couple of inches of space to be safe.

## TYPES OF JUICE FASTS

There are two basic versions of juice fasting: juice fasting with just juices, and modified fasting with juices and blended cold soups and green smoothies.

OPTION 1: **Vegetable juices only.** Make any of the vegetable juice recipes in this book or your own combinations. The vegetable-juice fast gets the best results; adding avocado, as recommended for smoothies and cold soups in option two, can slow the detox process. However, choose option two if you have low blood sugar, diabetes, extreme fatigue, or any other condition where you need to have some protein each day, unless your doctor advises you differently. Or you may want option two because you know that for emotional reasons, you would not fast otherwise. One option is to include wheatgrass juice twice a day. Drink about 2 ounces each time. There are people with hypoglycemia and even diabetes who have been able to do a short vegetable-juice fast when they've added the wheatgrass juice twice a day.

OPTION 2: **Juices, cold soups, and green smoothies.** A modified fast involves the use of fresh juices and blender smoothies. This fast allows you to have more substantial and calorie-rich liquids, as long as they're blended or pureed. I often make vegetable juice and put it into the blender with an avocado to make a thicker mixture with a smoothie-like consistency. The addition of the avocado will slow down the detoxification process, but the smoothie is still effective.

## What to Do During the Fast

**Drink plenty of purified water.** Be sure to get 2 to 2 1/2 quarts of water every day in addition to the juice. The more water you consume, the easier it is for your body to flush away the waste. Drinking enough water takes some discipline, but stick with it. Drink more than enough to satisfy your thirst. Keep drinking throughout the day.

**Include herbal tea.** You can include herbal tea in your plan. It is not a substitute for pure water, though. You will need your quota of water in addition to the herbal tea. Beneficial herbal teas include dandelion root and nettles, which help cleanse the liver and kidneys. Milk thistle is also extremely good for the liver. Peppermint is good for upset stomach, and chamomile is relaxing. You can also purchase detox teas in health food stores or supermarkets in the nutrition center. If you buy herbal tea in bulk, steep 1/2 to 1 teaspoon in a pint of hot water for ten minutes, strain, and drink warm. Lemon may be added for flavor, but do not use any sweetener, except a drop or two of stevia, if desired.

**Avoid stimulants.** Stay away from coffee, tobacco, alcohol, soft drinks, sweets, and all other stimulants. Most people can tolerate a small amount of white or green tea, but it should be on the weak side.

**Choose organic vegetables, herbs, and low-sugar fruit.** Some of the best vegetables and fruit for cleansing are carrots, beets, lemons, limes, sprouts of all kinds, wheatgrass, celery, kale, green peppers, cucumbers, parsley, asparagus, lettuce, spinach, collard greens, fennel, sweet potatoes, yams, garlic, ginger, grapefruit, and low-sugar apples like Granny Smith or pippin. Cabbage juice is also good, but it must be consumed immediately, as it does not store well. You will need a juicer that does wheatgrass juice if you plan to make your own. Or you can stop by a juice bar for a shot or two of wheatgrass juice each day. Make sure the wheatgrass is not sprayed to prevent mold. This is counterproductive to the whole cleansing process.

## Preparing Your Produce for Juicing

**Wash everything well, even if it's organic.** Organic produce is often still dirty and can have undesirable soil organisms or other contaminants on it. There are good vegetable washes available at health food stores and many grocery stores. You can also use sea salt in a sink full of water or food-grade hydrogen peroxide mixed in a basin of water.

**Prepare the produce for juicing.** Cut the produce into pieces that will fit into your juicer's feed tube. Peel the produce when appropriate; for example, remove grapefruit skin, which should not be consumed because of the volatile oils it contains. Slowly feed the pieces into the feeding tube. To juice leafy greens like spinach, parsley, lettuce, chard, or kale, bunch them up first, then push them through the juicer slowly with something hard like a carrot. Parsley works best if rolled up in a lettuce or kale leaf. When you have finished juicing, you can strain the juice if desired, then pour into a glass and drink.

**How to drink juice.** You can chill the juice if you wish, but drinking it at room temperature is easier on the digestive system. Be sure to swish the juice around in your mouth to mix with saliva, which is necessary for digestion of the carbohydrates in the juice. Try not to gulp your juice down too quickly; sip it slowly.

## What to Do During a Healing Crisis

Fasting can occasionally produce some negative symptoms because toxins are being moved out of storage places within the body and this release can cause some adverse symptoms. Detox symptoms are usually referred to as a healing crisis or the Herxheimer reaction. This crisis is good—it just feels bad sometimes, but it will pass; it's actually a good sign that you're getting rid of a lot of harmful stuff. Some possible symptoms include headaches; bad breath; a coated or furry tongue; canker sores; nausea, constipation, or diarrhea; skin eruptions; rashes; feelings of sadness, depression, or anger; backaches; muscle aches; light-headedness; weakness, tiredness, or fatigue. You may experience one or more of these symptoms as you juice fast, but don't worry, they'll soon pass.

During a healing crisis, there are several things you can do to help yourself feel better:

- **Take a short nap or a rest break.** Sleep more than usual during a fast.
- **Drink extra water,** fresh vegetable juice, or herbal tea to flush out the toxins.
- **Take extra vitamin C and magnesium citrate.**
- **Exercise** by taking a short walk, stretching, bouncing on a rebounder, or using a lymphasizer, all of which help the lymphatic system remove toxins more rapidly.
- **Take plenty of deep breaths.**
- **Take an enema or get a colonic** (see pages 151–54). Often, when you move waste out of the colon, all your adverse symptoms go away.
- **Use fiber** if you are constipated. Psyllium husks or flax fiber acts as a bulk laxative and can help move toxins through the colon more efficiently. Add 1 or 2 teaspoons of fiber to either juice or water, stir thoroughly, and drink immediately before it gets too thick. Use this three to five times a day during the first few days of a fast. Senna

tea is also helpful. (See other suggestions in chapter five, "Intestinal Cleansing for Vibrant Health.")

- **Dry skin brushing** is also good at this time, as it allows toxins to escape through the skin, which is the largest organ of elimination. Get a natural bristle bath brush and brush the skin in an upward motion.

- **Take a dry or infrared sauna** to sweat out more toxins. Sweating is the only way to get rid of plastic toxins.

- **Take care of your body and soul.** Rest, read a good book, call a fasting partner, meditate, or pray.

- **Give yourself positive self-talk.** Congratulate yourself for doing something great for your body. Tell yourself that you are getting healthier and more vibrant because of your efforts at fasting. If you don't feel as well as you'd like, tell yourself that this too shall pass. Remind yourself that on the other side is great healing, vibrant health, a trimmer body, and a renewed soul.

- **Remember that fasting is a choice that you made to help your body reach a higher level of health.** No one is making you do this; you chose it for yourself.

## Breaking the Fast

Breaking the fast is as important as the fast itself, and more important in some ways, in that if you break it with a big steak or a pizza, you could do your body harm and undo all the good you just did—and you could end up with a terrible stomachache. I know. Once, I broke my three-day juice fast with a salad from a restaurant salad bar and a few bites of seafood. But that was too much and I was doubled over in pain. Eat vegetables, seeds, a little low-sugar fruit, and some vegetable soups for a day or two after your fast and make sure to eat plenty of those foods raw. Chew everything well. Let your digestive system gradually return to normal. After the fast, the toxins that have been released may still be finding their way out through the channels of elimination, especially the colon, so it's best not to add too much food back into your diet right away, and certainly not heavy animal proteins that are hard to digest. Just as you resisted the temptation to have a last big supper before you began your juice fast, resist having a large meal soon after a fast.

Introduce heavy foods like proteins back into your diet slowly in small portions. You will probably find that you want less food, so now is not the time to go out with your friends to an all-you-can-eat buffet. If you go out for social or business reasons right after breaking your fast, you can ask for a special salad that has only vegetables, or get a vegetable soup or a vegetarian meal. Avoid the bread and butter. Order sparkling water or herbal tea with lemon or lime to drink.

### "How Do I Detox When I'm Busy?" and Other Frequently Asked Questions

Many people have asked me numerous questions through the years about how to make detox programs work for them. Here are some of the most often asked questions and answers:

**How do I fit detox programs into a busy schedule?** The best way to begin a detox program is on the weekend when you have a little more time to organize what you need. Prepare ahead for the workweek at this time. Most of the programs are just seven days, and you can get through nearly anything for a week. But you do need to be ready for the busy days by shopping in advance and preparing as much of the food as possible in advance. Remember, it's only seven days, but they are seven important days that could have a great impact on your health.

**Will I have low energy and not be able to do anything?** Most people find that their energy is not too low and they are able to do what they need to each day. But if your energy does become low, then take it easy. If you had a cold or flu, you'd probably have to slow down. The detox programs are very important for your health and will help you prevent colds and flus. If you have to take it a little slower for a few days, you're doing your body a big favor in the long run and it will reward you with greater energy in the future.

**Will the detox foods and supplements taste bad?** Most of the detox programs incorporate fresh juice, which tastes great. Many of the other recipes also taste good. A few herbal tinctures can have a strong taste. But nearly everyone is able to complete all the programs without a problem.

**How do I know if these programs are for me?** The detox programs are for everyone. We all need them because we're all bombarded with toxins in our air, soil, food, and water that interfere with our biochemical processes and contribute to weight gain, low energy, aging, sickness, and disease. Detoxing the body produces both immediate and long-term benefits.

**How do I tailor the programs to fit my schedule and needs?** First, try to pick a week when you don't have too many obligations, or move things around to free up more time. Prepare foods in advance to take to work. Let your family and friends know this is your week to take care of yourself and you won't be joining them for certain events or meals. If some parts of the program just seem impossible, do your best.

**What happens if I get off track?** As you detox your body, the important work of detoxification builds, day after day. If you cheat even one time in the middle, you'll either greatly slow the detox or stop it. You don't want to do that when you've worked hard to get to that place. However, if you do get off track, don't stop completely; keep going. You may want to add an extra day or two to your fast, depending on how far off track you got.

**How can I feed a family and stay on the program?** It may take some willpower if you have to make meals for your family and special

*(Continued)*

food for you. But you can do it. It's only for a week for most of the programs. If there's someone else in your family who can prepare meals during this time, it will help you a lot if they'd agree to make all the meals for the time you're on your detox program. Otherwise, prepare your food and theirs and eat your food while they eat theirs, maybe in different places. Think about what works for you.

**What if I have to do business over a meal during the detox?** You can order a big vegetable main-course salad without any animal products in it. Nearly every restaurant in America will prepare this kind of salad. You can ask for oil and vinegar for the dressing. You can order hot water and lemon or sparkling water and lemon or lime. This makes a great meal and may impress the people you are eating with. After all, you're eating really healthy, and most people wish they had that kind of willpower. If you're in the middle of a juice fast, you'll need to pass on the salad. Just explain what you're doing.

**What do I do at parties and during holidays?** You can drink sparkling water and lemon or just plain water, if need be. Most parties have a vegetable tray, so you can munch on the veggies. But make sure you eat what you need to before the party so you won't be hungry and tempted. Regarding holidays, it's best to avoid a detox program during major holidays. It's just too difficult for most people. But if you're battling a life-threatening illness, then you may want to embark on a detox program at this time so you won't be tempted to eat the wrong foods. For holidays that aren't major, this might be a time to do a detox program since you should have an extra day or two off from work when you can focus on your cleanse program and taking care of yourself.

**Which detox program should I start with?** I recommend you begin with the colon cleanse, then move to the liver/gallbladder cleanse, and finally the kidney cleanse. If you need any of the specialized cleanses, you can follow with those that apply to you. At any time, you can benefit from a one- to three-day vegetable-juice fast.

## Sample One-Day Juice Fast Guide

Below is a sample menu for a day of juice fasting. This menu can be modified or amended to suit your individual needs and tastes. You can choose any of these recipes or pick other recipes that suit your needs. You can follow this program for one, two, or three days, or more. If you're doing the modified juice fast, you can combine any of these juices with an avocado in your blender. This will make a great cold soup that is delicious and sustaining.

## BREAKFAST

### THE BREAKFAST ZINGER

*3 to 4 medium carrots*
*1 small beet with leaves*
*1/2 cucumber*
*1/2 small or medium lemon,*
    *peeled if not organic*

*1/2- to 1-inch piece fresh*
    *gingerroot*
*1/2 green apple (optional)*

Juice the carrots, beet, cucumber, lemon, and ginger. If you decide to use the apple, remember that it will add extra fruit sugar (avoid this if you are diabetic or hypoglycemic). Cut the apple into pieces and feed it into the juicer tube after the ginger. Stir the juice and pour it into a glass. Serve at room temperature or chilled.

## MIDMORNING BREAK

### THE WALDORF

*3 to 4 romaine lettuce leaves*
*3 organic celery ribs with*
    *leaves*
*1/2 cucumber*

*1/4 small or medium lemon,*
    *peeled if not organic*
*1/2 green apple (optional)*

Bunch up the lettuce one leaf at a time; push it through the juicer with the celery, cucumber, and lemon. If you decide to use the apple, remember that it will add extra fruit sugar (avoid this if you are diabetic or hypoglycemic). Cut the apple into pieces and feed it into the juicer tube. Stir the juice and pour it into a glass. Serve at room temperature or chilled.

## LUNCH

### SPINACH TOWER OF POWER

*1 to 2 cups organic spinach*
*1 handful parsley*
*3 to 4 medium carrots*

*1 organic celery rib with leaves*
*1/2 beet with stems and leaves*

Bunch up the spinach and parsley, and push them through the feed tube with the carrots, celery, and beet. Stir the juice and pour it into a glass. Serve at room temperature or chilled.

## HAPPY HOUR

### SOUTHWESTERN COCKTAIL

*1 medium vine-ripened tomato*
*1/2 medium organic cucumber*
*1/4 cup cilantro (use parsley if*
    *cilantro is too strong a taste*
    *for you)*

*1/4 small or medium lime or*
    *lemon, peeled if not organic*
*Dash of hot sauce (optional)*

Cut the tomato into sections that fit your juicer's feed tube. Cut the cucumber in half lengthwise. Bunch up the cilantro, and push it through the feed tube with the tomato, cucumber, and lime or lemon. Pour the juice into a glass, add the hot sauce (as desired), and stir. Serve at room temperature or chilled.

## DINNER

**Option 1:**
*Any of the juice recipes from chapter ten.*

## Option 2:

### CHERIE'S AWESOME ENERGY SOUP

Delicious and nourishing, this is a great recipe for those with hypoglycemia or diabetes.

| | |
|---|---|
| *4 to 5 medium carrots* | *1-to 2-inch piece of gingerroot,* |
| *1 cucumber* | *peeled if not organic* |
| *2 celery ribs* | *1 avocado, peeled, seed* |
| *1/2 lemon, peeled* | *removed* |

Juice the carrots, cucumber, celery, lemon, and ginger. Add the juice to a blender and then add the avocado. Blend until smooth. Pour the mixture into a bowl and eat with a spoon.

## BEDTIME SNACK

### SWEET DREAMS TONIGHT

| | |
|---|---|
| *2 romaine lettuce leaves* | *3 organic celery ribs with* |
| *1 handful parsley* | *leaves* |
| *4 carrots* | |

Bunch up the lettuce leaves and parsley, and push them through the feed tube with the carrots and celery. Stir the juice and pour it into a glass. Serve at room temperature or chilled, as desired.

---

#### Juicing Fasting for Life: Summary

Incorporate the vibrant health recommendations in chapter one for one to two weeks before the fast and follow the fasting guidelines.

**Step 1:** Eat whole, alkalizing, organic foods and eat 50 to 75 percent raw foods. Two days before fasting, increase to 75 to 80 percent raw.

**Step 2:** Remove as many sources of toxicity as possible.

**Step 3:** Drink plenty of purified water—2 to 2 1/2 quarts per day.
**Step 4:** Add fresh vegetable juices to your diet at least once or twice a day.
**Step 5:** Embark on a one- to three-day vegetable-juice fast.
**Step 6:** Break your fast wisely.

# CHAPTER FOUR

## Detoxing for Life

Thinking about our organs of elimination can be about as appealing as discussing how the clothes dryer's lint trap works or why the garbage disposal makes certain noises. But we all know these appliances are hot topics when they stop working efficiently or completely break down. The same is true for our organs of elimination. The trouble is, oftentimes we don't know they aren't working well; we just know we don't feel well.

A sound program of periodic detoxification will engage all the major organs in your body's detoxification system—intestines, liver, kidneys, skin, gallbladder, lungs, and lymphatics—to improve your health and prevent disease. You could consider detoxification as being like a thorough spring housecleaning that is taking place on the inside. Just as you need to deep-clean your home occasionally and really dig into corners, drawers, and closets where dirt and unwanted items accumulate, so you need to dig deeper when it comes to the organs of elimination and cleanse them thoroughly to eliminate the waste and toxins that have accumulated over time.

You could think of internal housecleaning in a creative new way: You have a good internal built-in vacuum system (the intestinal tract), a washing machine (the liver), lots of cleaning rags and fluids (the lymph and blood), a drain (the kidneys), a fan to blow out stale air and toxins (the lungs), and plenty of natural cleaning products (fresh juices loaded with antioxidants, herbs, and other supplemental nutrients) that will help you get the job done right.

The body is designed to detoxify a host of waste products. All you have to do is assist with the process by keeping out as many sources of toxins as possible while providing the right materials to assist in detoxification, such as good nutrition from juices, green smoothies, raw foods, and nutrient supplementation. And you can work on each of the major organs of elimination separately and in the right order— first the colon, then the liver and gallbladder, and finally the kidneys. Detoxing these primary organs of elimination will enable the supporting channels—the lungs, lymphatics, skin, and blood—to function at their maximum capacity.

It's estimated that on average people have at least 5 to 10 pounds of accumulated toxic waste in their cells, tissues, and organs. (That's 5 to 10 pounds we could really feel great about dropping!) Toxic substances that accumulate throughout the body can weaken and congest our organs and systems of elimination. As we've already seen, these substances come from a number of sources, such as the environment, unhealthy food choices, and internal by-products of metabolism, called endotoxins. Toxic substances such as chemicals, pesticides, drug residues, heavy metals, and food additives, along with by-products from food digestion, as well as yeasts, fungi, and parasites can pile up in our systems like logs jamming a river. If they are not broken down and eliminated, they are stored in the intestines, gallbladder, kidneys, liver, skin, bone, lymphatic system, and fat cells, making us sick, weak, overweight, and unable to fight off infections. In addition toxic molecules, known as free radicals, damage our cells, accelerating aging and creating many health problems. This is why it's so crucial to periodically cleanse your body.

The EPA reviews about 1,500 new chemicals each year. Thousands of different chemicals continue to pour into our environment, and we are exposed to thousands of toxins daily! Where do they go? More important, how do we get rid of them? The next two sections will give you a quick outline to help you understand how the body stores them, what happens with toxic buildup, and what your body does to detoxify and eliminate these toxins.

### Fighting the Free-Radical Battle

Free radicals are toxic molecules that bombard our healthy cells and cause damage. They are unstable molecules that have lost an electron, so they are quick to react with other compounds, trying to gain stability by capturing an electron from somewhere else. This sets off a chain reaction as the next molecule loses its electron and becomes a free radical itself. The process then begins to cascade, eventually resulting in the disruption of living cells.

*(Continued)*

The production of free radicals can be likened to the rusting of metal, which occurs when the metal reacts with oxygen in the air. This process is called "oxidation." The same thing happens inside us, as our bodies' molecules are also vulnerable to oxidation. This internal oxidation is what produces the free radicals that contribute to numerous health conditions, such as lack of energy and stamina, a less than optimal immune system, damaged cells, and premature aging.

Some free radicals are a normal result of biochemical processes and can easily be handled by our bodies' many defenses. However, nutritional and environmental factors such as pollution, radiation, pesticides, trans fats, and polyunsaturated fats in our diet can cause excessive free-radical activity that can cause damage.

Detoxification helps fight this free-radical battle in two important ways: first, by removing the source of excess toxicity and free radicals; and second, by contributing an abundant and powerful supply of antioxidants that attack the free radicals and neutralize them.

## Where Have All the Toxins Gone?

Toxins are a bit like criminals; they hole up anywhere they can find a place to hide. They hang out in cells, tissues, and organs. They can be found especially in fat cells and in the liver, kidneys, and large and small intestines. They hide in the mucous lining of the lungs and sinuses. And they are distributed into the cells and tissues of the brain, where they can cause a lot of cognitive and emotional problems. When the organs and systems of elimination get behind in their work, the toxins back up in the supporting systems just like dirty water backs up in a stopped-up sink. First the intestines build up mucus and putrefaction, and nutrients are not properly absorbed; then poisons are absorbed back into the bloodstream. The liver becomes overwhelmed and congested and our blood is not cleansed properly, so more toxins get into the bloodstream. The filtration system in the kidneys works hard to excrete toxic-laden urine, but they become overwhelmed, too, and some waste is recirculated.

This downward spiral affects more than just the elimination system. Toxins are shunted off to storage in fat cells so our organs will be protected from the acidity, since toxins are almost always acidic, and the body holds on to fat as a protection. Consequently, we have difficulty losing weight. These acidic pollutants collect in cells, tissues, and the fluids between the cells, making cellular metabolism inefficient at best. They can also show up as cellulite. And they can clog our skin, lungs, and the passages of the lymphatic system. The result of this toxic overload is sickness, tiredness, bad skin, and eventually disease.

### Flush Away the Cellulite

It's not just another fat. Simply put, cellulite is irregular fat deposits. Essentially, this fat is trapped within connective tissues and the affected areas are full of fluid, toxins, lymph, and waste. These dimples and bumps are usually found on the thighs, hips, and buttocks, and most people aren't very happy about them. Many dieters find that no matter how hard they work at weight loss, exercise, and strict diet, infuriatingly, this stuff sticks to the thighs like caramel on an apple—even when they've dropped a size or two.

Because it's quite different from your garden-variety kind of pudge, cellulite has to be tackled in a unique way. Cellulite is associated with poorly functioning blood vessels, constipation, poor lymphatic drainage, and toxicity. If blood vessels are weak and sluggish, toxins will accumulate quickly, making it difficult for the body to burn fat in the affected areas. Constipation contributes to cellulite because it causes wastes and toxins to remain in the body rather than being eliminated.

*(Continued)*

A sluggish, poorly functioning colon means that toxic wastes are not eliminated, and this affects the efficiency of organs such as the liver and kidneys.

Consuming sugar, refined salt (sodium chloride), caffeine, alcohol, tobacco, unhealthy fats and oils, and refined carbohydrates is taxing on your systems of elimination. This makes it much harder for your body to eliminate waste—and far easier for fat to get stored as cellulite. Some experts believe it's toxins that cause this fat to become trapped and held in one spot in the first place.

This kind of fat can't be eradicated just by eating healthy foods or by exercise. Though creams, lotions, or lymphatic drainage massage may help a little, they will not wipe away the lumps. You can rub, massage, and wrap this fat in seaweed every day of your life, but this stuff is not going to disappear unless you cleanse your body, especially your colon and liver, and improve your circulation and metabolism, get your lymph moving, and nourish your body from within. (One particular exercise machine known as a lymphasizer, or a swing machine, is particularly helpful; see the Resources Guide for more information.) Also, as you boost your metabolism, your circulatory and lymphatic systems will work better, and you'll increase your chances of shifting the bulges.

Changing your diet and detoxifying your body are key to eradicating cellulite. I know firsthand. You've got to flush out the toxins—plain and simple. It's also important to nourish and condition the areas affected in order to strengthen blood vessels and tissues and step up circulation. When toxins are removed and blood vessels and surrounding tissues are nourished, then it is possible for the fat to be used as energy. Your thighs don't have to look like a pitted golf ball any longer, and you can be trimmer *and sleeker* with the help of the cleansing programs.

## What Causes Toxic Buildup?

Environmental toxins from the air, soil, and water—substances such as pesticides, herbicides, industrial chemicals and solvents, ionizing radiation, and so many more—bombard us. Free radicals assault us further and weaken our ability to fight off viruses, bacteria, parasites, and cancer cells.

In addition, most people eat too much sugar, fast food,

junk food, and fried food; too many refined carbohydrates, such as white flour products; and too much food period, which overwhelms the body's capacity to keep up with the work of digestion, assimilation, and detoxification. Then we drink too much alcohol, take medications, and ingest too many chemicals, including preservatives, pesticides, and additives in commercial foods. Couple that with emotional toxicity such as fear, stress, worry, and anxiety, and we have a full-blown toxic overload.

Looking deeper at some of these toxic sources, we see things we don't tend to think about as being toxic, such as prescription and over-the-counter drugs. Pharmaceutical companies spend billions of dollars marketing drugs that frequently lead to side effects that are worse than the conditions they were meant to treat. These prescription and over-the-counter medications further contribute to a big toxic load on the liver that affects the entire body. The Centers for Disease Control and Prevention reports that poisoning from prescription drugs has become the second-largest cause of unintentional deaths in the United States. The *Times* analysis of 2009 death statistics showed that for the first time ever in the United States, more people were killed by prescription drugs than motor vehicle accidents; 37,485 people died from drug overdose, primarily from prescription pain and anxiety medications, versus 36,284 from traffic accidents. Drug fatalities more than doubled among teens and young adults between 2000 and 2008, and more than tripled among people ages 50 to 69.

It's important to avoid prescription and over-the-counter drugs as much as possible. When a doctor prescribes a medication, it's a good idea to get a second opinion, preferably from a doctor who specializes in natural medicine such as a naturopath or a holistic medical doctor. And always look up the side effects of that particular prescription before you take it. Look for a natural alternative remedy you can try first and lifestyle changes you can make to correct your health issues. This could make a huge difference in your health— both immediate and long-term.

Recently, I worked with a woman who had very high cholesterol. Her doctor wanted to prescribe cholesterol-lowering drugs, which she didn't feel comfortable taking. She opted for dietary changes and a red yeast rice supplement (rice that has been fermented by red yeast) under the supervision of a medical doctor. Within a short period of time her cholesterol went down to a healthy range and she was able to completely avoid drugs.

It's also important to avoid preservatives in our food. In 2006 the Food and Drug Administration (FDA) approved the spraying of viruses on all cold cuts to kill bacteria. The FDA has allowed refined food manufacturers to put "No Trans Fats" on the food labels if there is less than 0.5 gram per serving, so manufacturers have changed serving sizes to allow them to use this label. In small amounts, each of these additives may not sound like much, but added to all the other poisons we are exposed to daily, they place an incredible burden on our bodies' capacity to detoxify. Plus, no one has any idea about their interaction and what toxic by-products are created as a result.

The goal is to read labels and avoid everything with preservatives in it, as much as you possibly can. If you don't know what those strange-sounding words mean, don't buy that product. When the label says the product contains less than 0.5 gram per serving of trans fats, avoid it. This will mean that you avoid a lot of packaged and processed food and opt for much more fresh food.

### Sources of Toxicity

- Prescription drugs
- Additives from refined foods
- Aluminum and mercury from vaccines
- Mercury from amalgam fillings
- Biotoxins from mold or fungus
- Environmental toxins from paint, carpets, and new furniture
- Home cleaning products such as oven cleaners and toilet bowl cleaners
- Polishes for furniture and floors
- Air fresheners (sprays/solids)
- Antibacterial cleaners and soaps
- Dry-cleaning products
- Carpet and upholstery cleaners

## Do You Have Signs of Toxicity?

When the major organs of elimination—intestinal tract, liver, and kidneys—are not working properly, your blood becomes congested with chemical toxins, poisons, and other undesirable waste products. If these organs are clean and working efficiently, toxins will be filtered out and removed. When they remain in the body, they cause symptoms of toxic overload.

These symptoms are many and varied, and they affect people in different ways, depending on genetic makeup, weaknesses in certain organs, strength of the immune system, and emotional and mental states. For example, impure blood circulating through the brain can cause mental and emotional distress, depression, anxiety, and neurological diseases.

### Common Symptoms of Toxic Overload

- Lack of energy and fatigue
- Weakness
- Aches and pains
- Headaches
- Weight gain
- Inability to lose weight
- Irritability
- Emotional and mental problems
- Constipation
- Acid reflux
- Bloating and gas
- Indigestion
- Sinus problems
- Cellulite
- Trouble sleeping
- Restlessness
- Stressful feelings
- Dizziness
- Visual problems
- Skin problems
- Arthritis
- Hormone imbalances
- Premature aging

From the list of symptoms of toxic overload, you can see that it contributes to a host of ailments in our modern lives. For instance, constipation and acid reflux are problems that can be attributed to poor diet and toxicity, which affect many people. These conditions have become so prevalent that over-the-counter laxatives and antacids are among the most marketed drugs in this country. Chronic fatigue syndrome is another example of a condition that some doctors now believe is related to body toxicity. Many alternative medical doctors have found that cleansing the body of toxins is necessary to reverse this condition. (I'll attest to that firsthand;

read my story in the introduction.) Toxicity is also at the root of many other ailments we're suffering from in the United States, such as cancers, allergies, autoimmune diseases, yeast infections, stomach problems, multiple chemical sensitivities, and other environmental illnesses.

## Detoxification: Your Path to Vibrant Health

Your body uses amazing processes for removing toxic substances or transforming them into harmless by-products. It's something our bodies do as part of their normal functioning. Because the body is its own healer, detoxification is part of its normal function, like breathing or digestion. It clears out toxins by eliminating them through the colon, liver, kidneys, lungs, skin, lymph, and blood.

The idea of assisting the body in detoxification is not a modern invention. Cultures throughout history have practiced cleansing through fasting, the use of herbs, enemas, and various colon-cleansing practices. But only in the past few decades has detoxification become crucial for everyone who lives in a modern culture. There are just too many sources of contamination, toxicity, and chemical buildup to ignore their effects. In his book *The Detox Miracle Sourcebook*, Dr. Robert Morse says detoxification is "a system for removing the causes of disease, not a system of treatment or a way to remove symptoms. It involves the understanding that the body is the healer."

The detox programs in the next chapters will help you remove the causes of disease, and if you are ill, detoxing can help you restore your body to the balance it was meant to have. Your energy and vitality will be renewed, you'll lose fat and cellulite, stubborn symptoms will lessen or disappear, and you'll achieve the glow of health and vitality that may have been eluding you for a long time. The good news is that we have built-in processes for dealing with toxins, poisons, chemicals, yeasts, parasites, and internal by-products of metabolism. We just need to do our part by supporting our organs of elimination through cleansing.

**Benefits of Detoxifying**

- Weight loss
- Cellulite reduction
- Increased energy
- Fewer wrinkles and age spots
- Improved immune function
- Blood purification

- Neutralization and elimination of free radicals and other toxins
- Optimal digestive function
- Reduced cravings (e.g., for sugar, salt, junk foods, alcohol, and nicotine)

## The Organs of Elimination

There are five primary organs of elimination: the intestines, liver, kidneys, lungs, and skin. Additionally, there are three supporting channels: the gallbladder, lymphatic system, and blood. The colon, liver, and kidneys are the primary organs of elimination in the digestive system. These organs are responsible for expelling toxins, either by excreting them directly or neutralizing them so they are no longer toxic. The main way they are excreted is through the colon as feces and through the kidneys as urine. Meanwhile, the supporting channels, gallbladder, lymphatic system, and blood, help move the toxins and their by-products out of the body through bile, lymph, and blood.

The process breaks down when the intestinal tract becomes so clogged and congested that it is unable to properly eliminate waste. As you start the cleansing process, it's a good idea to first unclog these "pipes" with the colon cleanse. Next, cleanse and support the liver because it is the main organ of detoxification and is responsible for deactivating and removing toxic chemicals from the body. If it is compromised and weak, then it's unable to fulfill its proper role in detoxification, and toxins are stored away in places like that bumpy pudge on our thighs until the liver can get caught up again. Then cleanse the kidneys. And when you've completed your cleanses, you'll feel and look like a new person. Additionally, you can work on cleansing the lymphatic system, lungs, skin, and blood.

## THE FUNCTIONS OF THE DIGESTIVE SYSTEM

There are two main functions of the digestive system. The first part is digestion and absorption of food. The second part is elimination of waste. Here's an overview of the organs to help you understand what's going on.

**The Intestinal Tract: Your Internal Plumbing**

There are two main components of the intestinal tract—the small intestine and the large intestine, or colon. The intestines are coiled up inside the belly and stretch out to about twenty-six feet. That's a lot of surface area to allow absorption of nutrients and water to take place. More than 90 percent of all the nutrients we consume are absorbed in the small intestine, which makes it a key digestive organ.

**The Small Intestine.** The small intestine is made up of three segments: duodenum, jejunum, and ileum. The first section, the duodenum, is only about a foot or so long. This is where most of the minerals are absorbed from food. The next section is called the jejunum. It's longer—about eight feet. Here is where carbohydrates, protein, and water-soluble vitamins are absorbed. The final twelve-foot section is known as the ileum and is responsible for the absorption of fat, bile salts, cholesterol, and fat-soluble vitamins. Since the small intestine is responsible for extracting most of the nutrients from food, it's vitally important that it stay healthy and clean. Imbalances, congestion, and impaction of waste will interfere with its ability to sustain the body's nutritional needs. Many times people can eat reasonably well, yet they are not well nourished because of an improperly functioning small intestine.

**The Large Intestine.** The last five-foot portion of the intestine is known as the large intestine, or the colon. Food passes down this part of the digestive tract on its way to the anus, where it's excreted as feces. Along the way, it goes through three segments: the ascending colon, which connects to the end of the small intestine; then the transverse colon, which travels across the belly on top of the coiled-up small intestine; and finally, the descending colon, which heads down the left side of our bodies. At the very end, the descending colon attaches to the rectum, which holds the feces before sending it out through the anus.

When food comes out of the small intestine, it passes through a one-way valve called the ileocecal valve. It now enters the ascending colon, which is on the right side of the body. It's called "ascending" because it connects to the small intestine at a point toward the lower part of the abdomen, then moves up to the top of the coiled mass of the small intestine that is in the lower abdomen, transverses across the top, right to left, then descends down the left side. (This information may be helpful as you embark on the colon-cleansing program in the next chapter.)

As the semifluid ⋯ ⋯ moves on, it heads across the
t ⋯ l and some final nutrients are
e ⋯ ool is formed into a semisolid
s ⋯ as it travels along, gradually
g ⋯ rd the descending colon. The
st ⋯ o-thirds water, insoluble fiber,
a⋯ ird living and dead bacteria.
T⋯ lowest portion of the bowel,
w⋯ , and empties into the rectum
fo⋯

osal System. The colon, also

known as the bowel, is a crucial organ of elimination—it is our bodies' waste-disposal system. If it is not working properly, our health suffers. The primary job of the bowel is to get rid of waste and toxic materials. It moves this material through the intestinal tract by a process known as peristalsis, which is a kind of rhythmic wave of contraction. If all is going well, the food from the small intestine enters the colon within about eight to ten hours after being consumed. The colon is filled with billions of microorganisms, including friendly bacteria, yeast, and fungus, and although they live throughout the digestive system, most of them reside in the colon. A normal colon can contain as much as 4 pounds of these microorganisms. One type is known as "friendly bacteria," because they are friends of our bodies and necessary for the proper breakdown of proteins, as well as the synthesis of certain vitamins.

In addition to the friendly guys, the colon also has "neutral" and "unfriendly" bacteria. In a healthy person, there is a ratio of roughly 80 percent friendly and neutral bacteria to 20 percent unfriendly bacteria. The balance of good and bad bacteria can be disrupted by various factors, but particularly by the overuse of antibiotics and overconsumption of sweets. When the bacteria are out of balance and bad bacteria outnumber the good, the unfriendly opportunists begin to take over, producing too many endotoxins, which can be as toxic as most of the external toxins (exotoxins) from the environment.

These "bad" guys act on the undigested food in our guts, producing toxic chemicals and gases that can damage the mucous lining of the intestines, leading to intestinal toxemia. These potent chemicals include acetaldehyde, formaldehyde, alcohol, ammonia, skatoles, indoles, hydrogen sulfide, methane gas, carbon dioxide, and free radicals. Once the intestinal lining is damaged, it becomes more permeable, often causing a condition known as leaky gut syndrome. The unhealthy waste products can then leak out of the gut and get reabsorbed into the bloodstream, where they affect both our physical and mental health. Because these substances are extremely toxic, a bowel movement every eight to twelve hours—or two or three times a day—is ideal for good health. Most people in our society have far less than the ideal, which is a bowel movement after each meal.

Good bowel health is dependent on sufficient fiber and water in the diet so the stool can move freely through the intestines. The longer the stool remains in the intestinal tract, the harder it becomes, because water will continually be absorbed. A dehydrated stool becomes hard and compacted and is thus difficult to eliminate. Eating a poor diet that is low in fiber and water causes the feces to remain in the gut longer and longer. Also, being deficient in magnesium, vitamin C, or both can contribute to constipation. The longer the transit time, the greater the chance that the bad bacteria will overtake the friendly ones and the gut will become foul smelling and toxic. A strong-smelling stool or intestinal gas indicates increased fermentation and putrefaction (gas indicates that you may also need a liver or gallbladder cleanse or you're eating something you're allergic to).

The intestinal tract tries to protect itself from the constant exposure to toxic substances like drugs, environmental chemicals, food additives, refined carbohydrates (white flour acts like glue in the intestines), and heavy metals by creating mucus on the intestinal wall. As mucus builds up on the lining, toxins, yeasts, and parasites stick to it, until it becomes what is called "putrefactive debris." This substance can become hardened and rather rubbery in consistency. I've seen this firsthand. This prevents the proper assimilation of nutrients and contributes to toxins entering the bloodstream. This also creates a great space for parasites and yeasts to hide out.

In summary, the intestines feed our cells, tissues, and organs. If they are congested and contaminated, it will affect the health of our blood and lymph, causing them to be filled with impurities that are carried throughout the body and that the liver must filter. This is why a periodic program of cleansing for the bowel is so important to prevent waste from backing up into our entire systems.

**The Liver: Our Waste-Processing Plant**
Since the liver is the body's main organ of detoxification, we need it to be well functioning to survive this toxic planet. It works day and night filtering toxins, chemicals, and poisons from the blood, detoxifying anything that is dangerous to our systems, then neutralizing and eliminating those substances. It is the largest organ inside our bodies, weighing between 3 and 5 pounds, making it even bigger than the brain. It's

responsible for more jobs than any other organ—about five hundred in all. It's the busiest and hardest-working organ we have. If you put your hand on the right side of your abdomen, just under the diaphragm, you can feel it just slightly under the ribs. Think of it carrying out all these hundreds of vital functions and be thankful that it's working to keep you well, strong, and alive.

Every minute about 2 quarts of blood are delivered to the liver via the hepatic artery and the portal vein—that's about one hundred gallons of blood every day. This is an amazing figure, considering that our bodies have a total of about 5 quarts of blood in all. Oxygenated blood comes in from the hepatic artery, and deoxygenated blood comes from the portal vein, carrying nutrients that have been absorbed. The liver extracts life-giving nutrients and oxygen from the blood, as well as toxic chemicals and waste products. The nutrients are processed for energy, and the toxins are prepared for elimination. Richard Anderson, ND, author of *The Liver: Cleansing and Rejuvenating the Vital Organ*, says, "We cannot be healthy or recover from illness without a strong, clean, well-functioning liver. The life, health, and vitality of every single organ, gland, and cell are absolutely dependent upon the liver."

The liver becomes overwhelmed when it can't get rid of a lot of waste quickly enough. These toxic substances and waste products lodge in the cells and tissues, or they get shunted off for storage in fat cells. Colds, flu, rashes, skin eruptions and conditions such as eczema, headaches, bladder infections, and many other symptoms may develop as the body tries to maintain homeostasis by attempting to clean things out through the colon, skin, lungs, and kidneys. If we take drugs to suppress these symptoms, or cure a cold or flu, the toxins remain but are driven deeper into the tissues. Therefore, when we're sick, it's always best to treat our bodies with natural products and support our livers and immune systems. Drink lots of purified water and fresh vegetable juices along with herbal teas.

### The Liver's Important Jobs

Of all the important jobs that the liver performs every day, the following are the most important for maintaining health:

- Regulation of protein metabolism—necessary for hormones, enzymes, and structural components
- Regulation of carbohydrate metabolism and control of blood sugar—providing energy
- Production of bile—necessary for the emulsion and absorption of fats
- Making and breaking down hormones—needed throughout the body
- Detoxification of internal and environmental toxins—necessary for survival
- Filtering everything in the blood—nutrients, food, drugs, toxins, and alcohol
- Containing of cells, called Kupffer cells, which are part of the immune system—they tell the body about toxins in the liver

The liver's biggest and toughest job is detoxification, especially considering the enormous amount of material that assaults us daily. Try to imagine for a moment all the hundreds of chemicals and toxins floating through the blood waiting for cleansing and detoxification. It's like a line of hundreds of dirty campers waiting for the only shower in the campground. Yet these amazing livers of ours somehow manage to keep up the process. Nevertheless, the constant job of trying to detoxify all we put into our bodies can eventually overwhelm our livers, leading to health problems.

There are several hundred problems related to liver weakness. (See the "Symptoms of Liver Dysfunction" on pages 163–64 for a list conditions.)

## Kidneys: The Water-Filtration System

The kidneys are so important that we have two of them (some people are even born with three), although people are able to survive with just one. They are shaped like an ear and are purplish brown in color; each weighs about 5 ounces and measures about four to five inches long, three inches wide, and about one inch thick. They are situated at the back of the abdominal cavity, one on each side of the spine. The kidneys are made up of microscopic nephrons that are responsible for their functional and structural aspects and do most of their major work.

The outer portion of the kidney is called the cortex. It consists of capillary beds that filter the blood going to the nephrons that are located in the inner part of the kidneys. This is where filtration and reabsorption take place. The urine is formed inside the nephrons.

After the kidneys filter the blood, they return most of the water and many of the dissolved substances back to the bloodstream. What's left is called the urine, which passes through the ureters (tubular structures), then to the urinary bladder for storage, and finally through the urethra for elimination from the body.

**Functions of the Kidneys**

- Elimination of metabolic and toxic wastes
- Formation of urine from blood plasma
- Regulation of blood volume and blood pressure

- Regulation of ion levels in the blood
- Regulation of pH in the blood

The kidneys help excrete toxins via the urine. Some of these waste products, including ammonia and urea from the breakdown of amino acids, are the result of metabolism and are greatly increased with the consumption of excess animal products. Additional waste products include bilirubin from the breakdown of hemoglobin from the blood; creatinine from the breakdown of creatine phosphate in muscle fibers; and uric acid from the breakdown of nucleic acids. Also, many of the essential ions such as sodium, chloride, sulfate, phosphate, and hydrogen tend to accumulate in excess of the body's needs and must be eliminated. In addition, the kidneys excrete wastes from drugs, environmental toxins, and toxic substances from food and drink.

Kidneys are particularly sensitive to acidic wastes from such products as coffee, tea, soft drinks, chocolate, and alcohol. The overconsumption of acidic products can lead to kidney distress and may be felt as pain in the lower back.

Overconsumption of dairy products can lead to kidney stones, which are an accumulation of mineral salts combined mostly with calcium. The kidneys must handle all the excess toxicity that results when the liver and bowels are overwhelmed. The overconsumption of sugar and refined grains, salt, excess protein from animal products, and processed foods all put an additional burden on these organs.

## THE LUNGS AND RESPIRATORY SYSTEM: THE AIR-FILTRATION SYSTEM

The respiratory system comprises the nose, pharynx, larynx, trachea, bronchi, and lungs. We have a set of lungs that are situated in what's called the thoracic cavity, or chest. They are cone-shaped, spongy organs that are separated from each other by the heart. The right lung is thicker and broader than the left, as well as slightly shorter because the liver is on this side extending up into the diaphragm.

The lungs are considered one of the five major organs of elimination. Their function is to breathe in oxygen, hydrogen, nitrogen, and carbon from the air and process it by extracting what the body needs for fuel. Without oxygen the cells of our bodies cannot produce energy from the food we eat. This process is called cellular respiration. It involves the reaction of glucose from the breakdown of our food in the presence of oxygen, which then produces energy, with carbon dioxide as an end product. This cellular respiration occurs in each of the cells of our bodies. The lungs then expel carbon dioxide gas, along with some of the toxic waste processed by the body.

Inhaled oxygen and other gases are exchanged through small sacs called alveoli; then they move into the pulmonary capillaries of the lungs where they are sent to the heart, which pumps them to every cell in the body. The waste products of cellular respiration are then picked up and sent back to the lungs for exhalation. Along the way these expelled gases act as a filter for other toxins that we inhale, such as dust, chemicals, and gases. They are then picked up by the lymphatic system and the blood and are sent to the lungs to be exhaled. Other toxic substances are trapped by mucus in the lungs and are subsequently coughed up and spit out with the mucus.

## THE SKIN: THE CLEANUP CREW

Sometimes referred to as the third lung, the skin covers the entire surface area of our bodies, making it the largest organ of elimination. It is technically known as an organ because all of its tissues are structurally connected and it performs specific functions that benefit the entire body. One of these functions is to assist all the other organs of elimination in the process of detoxification, as well as acting as a barrier to prevent foreign or toxic substances from entering the body.

### The Five Major Functions of the Skin

- Protection from toxins, bacteria, dehydration, and UV rays
- Excretion of wastes, water, salt, and organic compounds
- Maintenance of body temperature
- Perception of stimuli
- Synthesis of vitamin D

Due to its large surface area, the skin can eliminate through its pores as much waste as the bowels, kidneys, and lungs together. This elimination is in the form of acidic toxins, gases, and mucus. If the colon, kidneys, or liver is backed up with toxic overload, the skin has to eliminate a larger part of the waste. If you are experiencing rashes, pimples, boils, acne, eczema, or abscesses, this indicates that your other organs of elimination may be unable to keep up with detoxification. As you detoxify, you may have skin eruptions, so don't be alarmed. Your body is working to get rid of toxins as fast as possible; these conditions will soon clear up.

## THE SUPPORTING CHANNELS OF DETOXIFICATION

The gallbladder, lymphatic system, and blood support the work of the primary organs of elimination.

### The Gallbladder: The Storage Tank

The gallbladder is a small pear-shaped organ located just under the right lobe of the liver. It's important in supporting the liver in eliminating toxins. The liver secretes toxins in a water-soluble form into the blood to be excreted by either the kidneys or the colon. It's transported from the gallbladder by bile, which is a carrier substance whereby many toxins are expelled from the body. A type of "holding tank" for the bile, the gallbladder stores and concentrates bile that is made by the liver until it's needed by the small intestine.

Bile is made up of bile acids, salts, cholesterol, and

electrolytes. It aids in digestion of fats. It's an alkaline substance that neutralizes stomach acid as the food comes out
of the stomach and heads for the small intestine. In the
meanwhile, the gallbladder stores bile until it gets a signal
to contract and release it. In the gallbladder, water and minerals are absorbed from the bile, and it becomes darker in
color, which produces a brown-colored stool. A light brown,
walnut-colored stool is a sign that the bile is a good quality.

## Lymphatic System: The Transport System

The lymphatic system is an arrangement of thin tubes that
runs throughout the body in the form of lymph vessels
and lymph nodes. They branch throughout the body like
the arteries except that they carry a colorless liquid called
lymph—a clear fluid that circulates around the body tissues
and contains a high number of lymphocytes (white blood
cells). Plasma leaks out of the capillaries to surround and
bathe the body tissues. This then drains into the lymph vessels. The lymphatic system also includes other organs—the
spleen, thymus, tonsils, and adenoids.

### The Lymphatic System Has Several Jobs

- Draining fluid back into the
  bloodstream from the tissues
- Filtering lymph
- Filtering the blood
- Fighting infections

The lymphatic system acts like a feeding station and drainage system for the cells of our bodies in that it carries nour-

ishment to the cells and transports away some of the waste. Our cells are a bit like babies: They eat, produce energy, excrete waste, and depend on us for their care. The cells are nourished by oxygen and nutrients from the blood, they metabolize these raw materials to generate energy, and then they dump the waste products out. The lymph system picks up some of the waste where lymph nodes and other lymphatic organs filter the lymph to remove microorganisms and other foreign particles, and lymphocytes destroy invading organisms.

Interstitial fluid is a watery substance that surrounds every cell in the body. It's the actual terrain that bathes the cells and picks up waste. It's particularly important to keep this fluid on the alkaline side by eating an alkaline-rich diet.

The lymphatic system is intimately connected to the immune system and carries out four major functions:

1. Draining excess interstitial fluid
2. Helping to maintain proper fluid balance
3. Transporting dietary lipids to the blood—fats and fat-soluble vitamins (A, D, E, and K) that are absorbed by the intestinal tract are transported to the blood
4. Carrying out immune responses—lymphatic tissue initiates highly specific responses directed against particular microbes or abnormal cells

It's important to keep in mind that the lymphatic system does not have an active pump like the heart but is instead moved by the skeletal respiratory pumps. Here's how it works: The skeletal muscles push against the lymphatic vessels, squeezing them in a type of "milking action." The respiratory system causes pressure changes that occur during inhalation—lymph flows from the abdominal region, where pressure is higher, to the chest area, where it is lower.

The health of the lymphatic system is tied to the health of the liver. If the liver is not properly detoxifying waste, more toxins will enter the lymph. It's therefore important to cleanse and detoxify the liver periodically, which will assist the entire lymphatic system in its important work of carrying toxins out of the body.

## Blood: The River of Life

Blood is called our "river of life" for good reason; it brings life-giving nutrients such as oxygen, vitamins, and minerals to the trillions of cells in our bodies, then carries waste to the organs of elimination. Blood is actively pumped throughout the body by the heart.

### Functions of Blood

- Regulation of pH—acidity or alkalinity (blood must be maintained at about 7.35 to 7.45 on the pH scale)
- Regulation of body temperature—normal is approximately 98.6°F
- Regulation of the water content of cells
- Transportation of oxygen and nutrients to the cells from the lungs
- Transportation of carbon dioxide to the lungs
- Transportation of waste products from the cells to the liver, kidneys, lungs, and sweat glands for expulsion

## Cleanse and Renew

Cleansing each of the organs of elimination is crucial if we want to have abundant health. We have seen the many ways toxins can accumulate in our organs of elimination. It's the accumulation of these toxins that keeps many people in a place of "dis-ease," where they often feel sick and tired. To prevent illness and enjoy optimal health, it's imperative to get rid of the buildup of waste throughout the body by removing toxins, drug residues, heavy metals, acid, parasites, fungi, yeasts, and other pathogens. As you detoxify your organs and systems of elimination, you'll begin to feel better—perhaps better than you've felt in years. Cleansing will give you an amazing sense of well-being, energy, and life! Plus, it will help you prevent disease. Your reward will be a life of abundant health and the energy to fulfill your purpose.

The programs that follow in the next chapters have succeeded for me and for countless numbers of people whom I've worked with through the years. The elimination of wastes and toxins will facilitate weight loss, oftentimes where nothing else may have worked. People often exclaim that their excess weight just melted away! Cellulite, which is trapped toxins, water, and fat cells, usually improves or goes away completely.

Adding a detoxification program can dramatically change your health and give you a more youthful appearance. I encourage you to stick with these cleansing programs until you have systematically detoxed each major organ or system in your body. You will be rewarded with high-level wellness. And then, just like you maintain your car, you need to cleanse your organs at least once a year.

**Detoxing for Life: Summary**

Step 1:  Eat whole, alkalizing, organic, non-GMO foods; remove as many sources of toxicity as possible; drink plenty of purified water, and eat 50 to 75 percent of your food raw.

Step 2:  Add fresh vegetable juices to your diet at least once or twice a day.

Step 3:  Complete a one- to three-day juice fast.

Step 4:  Complete the colon, liver and gallbladder, and/or kidney cleanse programs.

# CHAPTER FIVE

## Intestinal Cleansing for Vibrant Health

While colon cleansing is far from a sexy subject, the results it achieves are truly exciting. It's one of the most effective keys for weight loss and great health.

Whether you call it the large intestine, bowel, or colon, the reality is that for a lot of us, it's congested. Actually, the entire intestinal tract can become congested. A thorough cleansing of the whole intestinal track is a great way to boost your energy and vitality and overcome some common symptoms of ill health, such as poor digestion, constipation, acid reflux, stomach pain, irritable bowel syndrome, *Candida albicans*, gas, bloating, protruding belly, headaches, and low energy. And if you want to lose weight quickly and easily, it's crucial to cleanse the intestinal tract.

Intestinal cleansing is one of the most important steps— and usually the most overlooked—when it comes to losing weight, reshaping the body, flattening the abdomen, improving digestion and elimination, and restoring health. The problem is that we can't properly digest and eliminate food and substances we ingest when the colon is congested. The more congested it is, the more waste in the forms of old fecal matter and mucus can lodge in the lining. People can end up carrying around pounds of this stuff. Not only does this interfere with the normal two to three bowel movements per day needed for good health, but it also interferes with nutrient absorption from our food and supplements.

Combining colon cleansing with a good weight-loss diet, such as the Juice Lady's Turbo Diet or the Coconut Diet (programs for effective weight loss), can help you trim your waistline faster and more completely than any diet by itself. A stomach that protrudes may not be just from fat; it can also be the result of intestinal waste buildup. When the entire intestinal tract is cleansed, the stomach often flattens. The colon can also function better, eliminating wastes quicker, which greatly facilitates weight loss and boosts health. And nutrient absorption is improved so your body is better fed. As a result, cravings usually diminish or disappear, making it easier to stick with your healthy lifestyle program.

It's always a good idea to begin a detox with a thorough cleansing of the bowel before you move on to other organs. When your body detoxifies, it dislodges poisons and toxins that have built up in cells and tissues. Your body will pull toxins out of all their hiding places. These wastes are then deposited in the colon for rapid elimination, but if it's congested with old fecal matter, then the toxins can't skip on out as easily. They'll just sit around and get reabsorbed back into the bloodstream. And you could experience more headaches, weakness, fevers, chills, nausea, skin eruptions, and other detox symptoms.

## The Root of Many Health Problems

A congested colon is at the root of numerous health problems. Some natural healing professionals believe it's the principal cause of nearly every disease. Considering we spend seven hundred to eight hundred million dollars a year in this country on laxatives, it's fair to say that many Americans have sluggish, constipated bowels. Dr. Bernard Jensen was a pioneering chiropractor and nutritionist who began his career in 1929 writing about proper bowel management. His books are still considered classics in the field of detoxification. Dr. Jensen states that "in the fifty years I've spent helping people to overcome illness, disability and disease, it has become crystal clear that poor bowel management lies at the root of most people's health problems."

### Clogging Versus Cleansing Foods

| CLOGGING (COLON-UNFRIENDLY) | CLEANSING (COLON-FRIENDLY) |
|---|---|
| • Refined flour products (e.g., bread, pasta, pizza dough, bagels)<br>• Cheese<br>• Other dairy products | • Vegetables (especially high water content)<br>• Fresh vegetable juices<br>• Fresh whole fruit |

(Continued)

| CLOGGING (COLON-UNFRIENDLY) | CLEANSING (COLON-FRIENDLY) |
| --- | --- |
| • Meat<br>• Trans fats<br>• Sweet treats and desserts<br>• Snack foods (potato chips, corn chips, bagel chips, cheese puffs, etc.)<br>• Fast foods (French fries, burgers, tacos, deep-fried foods) | • Whole grains (e.g., brown rice, quinoa, barley)<br>• Legumes (beans, split peas, lentils)<br>• Flaxseeds (ground)<br>• Most nuts (soaked in water or ground are best)<br>• Fresh herbs (e.g., parsley, cilantro, basil)<br>• Filtered or purified water<br>• Herbal teas<br>• Fiber supplements |

## What Happens When the Colon Doesn't Work Efficiently?

The following points will help you better understand what is going on in the intestinal tract when it's not functioning well:

◆ The feces become dehydrated and compacted in the colon, leading to constipation, which many health professionals believe contributes to disease.

◆ Old fecal matter and sticky mucus can become lodged in or stuck to the sides of the intestinal tract, which leads to an irritation of the lining of the colon.

◆ Pathogenic organisms like bacteria, viruses, parasites, and yeasts such as *Candida albicans* are able to proliferate in a toxic colon. These pathogens excrete waste material in the form of toxic enzymes, acids, and gases that cause inflammation and eventual degradation of the intestinal walls.

◆ When the feces are moving too slowly through the bowel, the toxins have more time to penetrate the bowel wall and move into the bloodstream.

◆ Recirculating toxins cause weakness in tissues and organs throughout the body.

◆ Toxins accumulate in our cells, tissues, blood, and organs such as the colon, liver, and brain and stay there, causing numerous health problems.

◆ The immune system becomes overwhelmed with the toxic overload as white blood cells take up toxic debris. This leaves us vulnerable to a host of diseases.

## Symptoms of a Toxic Colon

Digestive health can suffer as a result of toxic overload in the colon and can lead to seemingly unrelated problems like skin conditions, joint pain, sinus problems, varicose veins, forgetfulness, and irritability, to name just a few. A malfunctioning colon is at the root of hundreds of illnesses and diseases.

Often people think their health concerns have nothing to do with the colon because they are manifested somewhere else in the body. For example, an impacted colon can press against nerves and cause back pain, sciatica, and leg pain, since it's close to the nerves from the spine; or an impacted colon can release toxins that travel to other parts of the body, causing headaches and sinus infections. You may have a bowel movement every day, but that does not mean your colon isn't congested.

---

### Symptoms of a Toxic Colon

The following symptoms are often associated with a congested colon. You may not have all these symptoms; actually, you may have just a few of them. This may still indicate the need to detoxify or cleanse your intestinal tract.

- Chronic constipation
- Gas and bloating
- Diarrhea
- Weight gain and inability to lose weight
- Low energy or fatigue
- Impaired digestion
- Stomach pain
- Irritable bowel syndrome
- Leaky gut syndrome
- Acid reflux or heartburn
- Diverticulitis
- Crohn's disease
- Swollen or protruding belly

- *Candida albicans* (yeast infection)
- Parasites
- Food allergies
- Gluten sensitivity
- Lactose intolerance
- Hemorrhoids
- Irritability, mood swings
- Foul-smelling stools or gas
- Frequent colds
- Chronic headaches
- Rashes, skin eruptions
- Colon cancer

---

## Common Problems of the Colon

Following are common bowel problems that plague millions of Americans. These conditions can be greatly improved with a colon detoxification program.

## CONSTIPATION

Constipation refers to difficulty or infrequency in passing stools. Constipation can undermine the health of the whole body, affecting digestion, preventing a clearing of toxins, lowering energy levels, and hindering efficient absorption of nutrients.

Poor diet is a major contributor to constipation, as is poor liver function, parasites, *Candida albicans*, and low thyroid function, along with deficiencies in nutrients such as magnesium and vitamin C. Food allergies and sensitivities can also be contributing factors. Too much dairy and refined grains can be quite constipating. And stress has an adverse effect on the colon—indeed on all the organs.

The treatment of constipation includes adequate fiber, plenty of water, sufficient vitamin C and magnesium, improvement in thyroid health, exercise, and *Candida albicans* and parasite cleansing, along with colon and liver cleansing. When you cleanse the intestinal tract, constipation is usually alleviated and weight loss becomes easier. Drinking fresh vegetable juices can also be very helpful, since they supply a good source of soluble fiber, which is very beneficial to the colon.

## COLON CANCER

Colon cancer, or colorectal cancer, involves cancerous growths in the colon, rectum, or appendix. More people die each year from colorectal cancer than from breast cancer and AIDS combined. After lung cancer, it is the leading cause of death from cancer in both men and women. It's the third-most-diagnosed cancer in the United States and Canada (excluding skin cancer). Only lung and breast cancers in women, and lung and prostate cancers in men, are diagnosed more frequently.

Studies show that a diet high in red meat and low in vegetables, fruit, and other high-fiber foods contributes to an increased risk of colon cancer. The best preventive program is one that includes reducing clogging foods, eating more cleansing foods, drinking more water, exercising, and completing periodic colon cleansing, along with periodic preventive testing for those at high risk or over fifty.

## DIVERTICULOSIS OR DIVERTICULAR DISEASE

The latest statistics reveal that the number of Americans who suffer from diverticulosis is increasing. The National Institute of Diabetes and Digestive and Kidney Diseases reported that 10 percent of Americans over forty have diverticulosis. By age sixty the figure jumps to 50 percent. The good news is that proper care of the colon can prevent this condition or keep it from developing into the more serious form known as diverticulitis.

Diverticulosis is a condition that results when small pouches called diverticula form in the colon. These pouches bulge outward through weak spots in the colon wall. If they become infected, the condition is called diverticulitis. Diverticular disease is believed to be caused principally by a low-fiber diet that leads to constipation. The resulting pressure on the colon wall causes a diverticulum to form. It's interesting to note that diverticular disease was not even observed in the United States until the early part of the 1900s, when low-fiber, processed foods were first introduced into the American diet.

## Contributors to Poor Colon Health

In addition to poor diet, lack of exercise, insufficient fiber, and not drinking enough water, there are a number of other factors that contribute to poor colon health, including stress, an imbalance of good and bad bacteria, inadequate chewing of food, overeating, and improper food combining.

Toxic emotions such as fear, stress, worry, and anxiety take a particular toll on the digestive system. The autonomic nervous system controls all unconscious activity in the body, including control of the digestive system. When it's stressed, the nervous system diverts energy away from the digestive organs and routes it to the musculoskeletal system to mobilize us for action in what is known as the "fight-or-flight" response. During this stress reaction, the intestines and kidneys slow down so the body can use the energy to run away or fight the enemy. The problem with our fast-paced lifestyles is that we perceive threat on a continuous basis, and our digestive systems suffer continually. Stress also decreases saliva flow and lowers the output of digestive enzymes and hydrochloric acid. A stressful lifestyle results in impaired digestion and decreased bowel function. To help your digestive health, it's best not to eat when emotionally upset, angry, or worried until you can calm down and let your body return to a state of balance.

## IMBALANCE OF GOOD AND BAD BACTERIA

A healthy intestinal tract has a complex ecology of friendly, neutral, and unfriendly (pathogenic) bacteria. An overgrowth of unfriendly bacteria, yeasts, and parasites can disrupt the delicate balance of the entire gastrointestinal tract. This overgrowth eventually leads to inflammation in the sensitive mucous lining, which then interferes with the proper assimilation of nutrients.

The contributing factors to imbalanced intestinal flora include a diet that is high in animal muscle meats and fats, trans fats, processed foods, low-fiber foods, sugar, coffee, tea, and alcohol, as well as overuse of antibiotics, over-the-counter drugs like acetaminophen and aspirin, plus a diet that lacks essential nutrients. Antibiotics are particularly damaging to this delicate balance because not only do they kill the bacteria they were prescribed for, but they also destroy friendly bacteria in the colon. The good bacteria have many beneficial functions, such as converting certain raw materials into much-needed nutrients. They're also responsible for keeping pathogenic bacteria and yeast that live in the colon in check. Once this delicate balance is disrupted, the unfriendly bacteria begin to outnumber the good, which causes more toxins to be released. Additionally, yeasts rapidly proliferate, causing more problems because *Candida albicans* releases numerous toxins into the body, including acetaldehyde and ethyl alcohol.

A typical American diet that is high in bad fat and refined carbs, especially flour products, and low in fiber has a tendency to stick to the inner walls of the intestinal tract and results in an impacted layer developing in the intestines. This condition eventually leads to a buildup of mucus, which decreases the available binding sites for the good bacteria. Removing this toxic-laden mucous layer through colon cleansing enables the friendly bacteria to attach to the intestinal walls again and helps restore the balance of intestinal flora. Use of a good probiotic formula will reintroduce friendly bacteria such as *Lactobacillus acidophilus* and *Lactobacillus bifidus* into the colon.

## Simple Tips for Optimal Digestion

Are you one of those busy people who eat meals on the run? Many people get so hurried with their busy schedules that they grab something quick and easy, barely chew it, and then wash it down with a big gulp of a soft drink, iced tea, or water. If this describes you, you may have noticed that your digestion is not as good as it used to be. Most of us can get away with this to some degree when we're young, but the older we get, the more our digestion becomes challenged by a hurried lifestyle. One of the best ways to help your digestion improve is to slow down, take a few breaths, say a thanksgiving for your food, and slowly begin chewing thoroughly. Instead of thinking "fast food," start thinking in terms of "slow food" eating. Set aside enough time in your schedule to do nothing but eat, preferably enjoying your food with family and friends as often as possible, the way many Europeans do.

Digestion actually begins in the mouth. First we chew our food, breaking it down into smaller and smaller particles. As we chew, saliva mixes with the food and starts the process of digestion. Saliva contains the enzymes ptyalin and amylase, which begin digestion of the carbohydrates in vegetables, fruit, starches, and sugars in the mouth. Other enzymes act on any bacteria that might be in the food, thereby providing the first line of defense against foreign invaders. Not taking the time to properly chew your food interferes with this initial digestion process and can lead to many problems, such as indigestion, acid reflux, leaky gut syndrome, and constipation.

Your mother was right when she said, "Chew, chew, chew your food!" You need to chew each mouthful at least twenty to thirty times before you swallow it. Follow the adage "Chew your juice and juice your food." Insufficient chewing puts stress on the digestive system because food particles that are not broken down well enter the intestines, where they can produce toxic metabolites that leak through the membranes in the intestines.

Limit the amount of water you drink with meals, and especially limit ice-cold liquids, because they can interfere with proper digestion. Too much liquid with meals dilutes the digestive enzymes in the mouth and the stomach, so the food is not properly digested, leading to many of the problems we've been discussing. The stomach contains hydrochloric acid, which acts on proteins, denaturing them and preparing them for the next stage of digestion. The stomach also contains a protein-digesting enzyme called pepsin and a fat-digesting enzyme known as lipase. Drinking too much liquid with your meals makes it difficult for these enzymes to work efficiently, so food enters the intestines in a partially undigested state. Try to drink no more than 4 ounces of liquid with your meals, preferably at room temperature. The best approach is to stop drinking lots of liquids about half an hour before meals, and then resume at least a half hour after.

To improve your digestion, you may also need digestive enzymes. I like a particular type of enzyme that is taken between meals that cleans up undigested particles of food that were not broken down. It helps a lot with hair growth. (See the Resources Guide for more information.) Also, as we age, beginning at about age thirty-five, the production of hydrochloric acid slows down. We can benefit by taking a supplement called betaine hydrochloride. You'll notice a difference; your nails will grow longer and stronger.

## Overeating

In these days of supersize meals, most people have become accustomed to eating far too much food. Americans have been programmed by the food industry to eat, eat, eat, but the sad news is that overeating causes more health problems than just about anything else. Even eating too much healthy food puts a strain on the digestive system and can lead to problems such as obesity, high blood pressure, heart disease, acid reflux, and constipation.

Many studies have shown that people who habitually undereat live longer and are healthier than their overeating counterparts. Calorie restriction helps improve health and slows the aging process. Smaller portions support digestive health. We can be particularly watchful when eating out. For example, instead of heaping food on our plates from a buffet, we can choose a reasonable serving. In restaurants that serve large portions, we can share a dinner with a friend or ask for a take-home carton. One easy rule of thumb is to eat only half as much as you are accustomed to. You'll be surprised at how quickly your body adapts to smaller portions. And your waistline will reap a big reward!

## Improper Food Combining

There are many theories about how to combine food for maximum digestive health, and a certain amount of disagreement exists among health practitioners. Nevertheless, there are a few standards that almost everyone agrees on. The most important rule is not to mix heavy-protein foods such as meat with starchy carbohydrates such as potatoes or refined carbohydrates such as bread and pasta. This teaching challenges the tradition of hamburgers and sandwiches, meat and potatoes, and spaghetti and meatballs that are so popular in our culture. This is not to say that you can't ever have such a meal again, but work on having them less often. The problem is that proteins require different digestive enzymes than carbohydrates. If you have digestive challenges, try eating your protein with only vegetables, and especially include some high-water-content foods like leafy green vegetables. A big salad, a steamed vegetable, and a small piece of free-range poultry or fish make an ideal alternative to meat, potatoes, and bread. If you choose to have a meal of grains rather than protein, use whole grains like brown rice, quinoa (pronounced *keen-wa*), millet, or spelt combined with lightly steamed vegetables and a big salad. This way of eating not only is more conducive to good digestive health, but also is the way to maintain a good alkaline balance—one of the pillars of a healthy eating program.

## The Goal of the Colon-Cleansing Program

Completing a colon cleanse will help you improve digestion and colon health. By eliminating waste that's stuck in the large intestine, you create a better environment for evacuation. Also, colon cleansing increases the colon's ability to absorb essential nutrients and water. The result will be a better-nourished body.

"What is a normal bowel movement?" people frequently ask. It's surprising how many people think normal is to have one bowel movement every other day, or even less often. For some, it's once a week. Health researchers have studied people who live in nonindustrialized, rural communities, who eat a simple, natural, whole foods diet and get a moderate amount of exercise. They've determined that these people set the standard for a healthy colon. You might be surprised to learn that they will have a bowel movement within about a half hour after eating a meal, which means that their bowels move two to three times a day. Two to three times a day should be our goal. And yes, it's possible to reach this goal once the colon is cleansed and restored to health.

Another question people frequently ask is "What does a healthy bowel movement look like?" Healthy feces will be walnut brown in color, will appear soft and unformed, with about the consistency of peanut butter, and will float for a moment before slowly sinking as they begin to break up. They will not be hard, dark in color, pencil thin, or a series of hard pellets. By this definition, there aren't too many people in America who can report that their colons are working efficiently most of the time.

The goal in the colon-cleansing program is to remedy poor colon health by restoring normal muscle movement in the intestines (peristalsis) so the waste that is inhibiting digestion and assimilation can be removed. The colon-cleansing program will require some time and effort for a week or two, but the rewards are well worth it. If we cooperate with our bodies, and cleanse our colons, they will heal and function normally again.

### The Colon Detoxification Program

A thorough detoxification program includes these six important steps:

1. Reduce exposure to toxins—from the environment or from processed foods.
2. Eat a health-building diet—with plenty of vegetables and fresh vegetable juices.

3. Eliminate coffee, alcohol, nicotine, and over-the-counter medications.
4. Exercise—sweat to eliminate toxins.
5. Drink plenty of water to flush toxins.
6. Detoxify your colon.

## The Colon-Cleanse Program

During the colon-cleanse program, you can eat two to three meals a day, but they should be light and healthy, mostly raw with plenty of raw vegetables, vegetable juices, and some low-sugar fruit such as berries or green apples. For maximum results, you could start your program with a three-day vegetable-juice fast. Some recommend just drinking apple juice, but apple juice contains too much fruit sugar, so I don't recommend this method.

During the colon cleanse you will be drinking and eating lots of colon-cleansing, alkaline foods like high-water-content leafy green vegetables and brightly colored vegetables, plenty of fresh vegetable juices, green smoothies, fresh whole fruit, and ground raw seeds and nuts. The cleanse works best when you avoid heavy animal foods like meats, cheese, and other dairy products and processed grains such as bread and pasta. You can have an egg or a little fish, but I recommend limiting them as much as possible for maximum colon cleansing. You can have any of the colon-friendly foods listed in the box on pages 129–30, but limit whole grains and legumes to a small amount once a day.

## MENU PLAN

**Upon Rising**

> **7:00 A.M.** Drink the Fiber Shake or Toxin Absorber Shake (see
> suggestions on pages 147–48 or the Resources Guide).

**Breakfast**

> **8:00 A.M.** Choose one of the following:

> 1. Awesome Green Smoothie with ground almonds, or
> 2. Avocado and sliced tomatoes, or
> 3. One of the vegetable juice recipes in chapter ten.

> **9:00 A.M.** Take a probiotic.
> **10:00 A.M.** Drink fresh vegetable juice such as the Colon
> Cleanse Juice Cocktail or any juice recipe.
> **11:00 A.M.** Have a Fiber Shake or Toxin Absorber Shake.

**Lunch**

> **12:00 Noon** Choose one of the following:

> 1. Large mixed vegetable salad and a cup of raw soup
>    (see recipes starting on page 319), or
> 2. Large mixed vegetable salad with avocado (be
>    creative and add lots of different vegetables) and
>    1/2 cup cooked brown rice (or other whole grains
>    such as quinoa or millet), or
> 3. Chopped hearty vegetable salad—bite-size pieces of
>    broccoli, cauliflower, red and green pepper, celery,

cucumber, radishes, tomato, yellow squash, and
zucchini; add some sprouted alfalfa or sunflower
seeds, cilantro, or parsley for variety.

Salad dressing favorite: Shake 1/2 cup extra-virgin olive
oil, 3 tablespoons Bragg Liquid Aminos (a liquid protein concentrate available at health food stores), 3 tablespoons lemon
juice, and 3 tablespoons water together in a glass container
and add herbs of your choice and fresh minced garlic or
ground garlic to taste.

   **4**. Fresh vegetable juice (your choice)

## Afternoon
   **3:00 P.M.** Have a Fiber Shake or Toxin Absorber shake.
   **4:00 P.M.** If you're hungry, choose a juice or smoothie recipe or
      low-sugar fruit like berries or a green apple.

## Dinner
   **6:00 P.M.** Prepare a dinner that follows the healthy guidelines.
      Use one of the lunch suggestions, or be creative with
      vegetable dishes. If you are doing three days of juice
      fasting, then choose a vegetable juice recipe. Be sure to
      include plenty of raw vegetables such as a salad, sliced
      tomatoes, vegetable sticks, or lightly steamed vegetables
      like broccoli, asparagus, Brussels sprouts, carrots, and
      onions. You may add 1 or 2 ounces of chicken, turkey,
      or fish if you really have to have more protein, but
      remember that animal products are clogging as opposed

to cleansing, so it's best if you can omit them. Your cleanse will proceed more quickly if you skip all animal protein. You will not lose muscle mass while forgoing animal protein for a week or two.

**After Dinner**

Take an herbal cleanse formula. Herbal colon-cleanse products must be purchased. Take according to manufacturer's directions; usually one or two capsules are sufficient (see the Resources Guide).

**8:00 P.M.** Drink herbal tea and take a probiotic.
**9:00 P.M.** Have a Fiber Shake or Toxin Absorber Shake.

## DURING THE CLEANSE

During the cleanse you will have four to five fiber shakes a day, plus an herbal cleansing formula at least once a day, usually with or right after dinner. Continue to drink plenty of water between meals, aiming for 2 to 2 1/2 quarts per day (there are four 8-ounce glasses per quart, so that's eight to ten glasses a day). Also, you may drink herbal tea throughout the day and count it toward your water quota. You can sweeten drinks with a little stevia, but don't use sugar or honey. Early in the day it's fine to have one or two cups of green tea or white tea, both of which contain some caffeine, though not as much as coffee, but avoid them later in the day or if you tend toward low blood sugar or poor adrenal function.

## Fiber Shake

When you're not juice fasting, you'll want to eat a high-fiber diet during this program, as well as on your maintenance program. You'll also add additional fiber and bentonite clay as part of the cleanse in order to facilitate the movement of impacted waste from the colon. The fiber acts like a broom to sweep the walls of the colon, and bentonite clay acts like sponges to soak up toxins and waste material so they can be eliminated.

Bentonite is a type of clay composed primarily of montmorillonite or other minerals. It is derived from volcanic ash, and there are two major commercial varieties—sodium bentonite and calcium bentonite. Sodium bentonite is readily absorbent and swells in the presence of water. Calcium bentonite's structure, on the other hand, does not permit it to expand when liquid is added. Both types of bentonite are effective binding agents.

The colon-cleanse products used may include flax fiber, or ground flaxseeds, bentonite clay, apple pectin, and a small amount of ground psyllium husks or seeds. Adding activated charcoal helps absorb even more of the toxins as they are released.

There are a number of products available. I like Toxin Absorber, which is psyllium seed husk, bentonite clay, apple pectin, and peppermint leaf or ginger (see the Resources Guide). You can mix your own, but many people have told me it is not easy to find the right ingredients.

Nevertheless, if you want to try this, you can consult the recipe in the following section. Many commercial products principally contain psyllium husks or seeds, which in large amounts can cause bloating or constipation in some people and may be too drying for your colon. But a small amount mixed with other fiber usually works quite well. I don't recommend wheat bran since so many people are sensitive to wheat; alternatives include oat bran and rice bran. Read labels carefully before purchasing a product (see the Resources Guide).

## HOMEMADE FIBER BLEND

Most of the products listed here are available in your local health food store or natural foods store. You may also want to purchase a seed grinder or a small inexpensive coffee grinder so you can grind your own flaxseeds.

*1/2 cup flax fiber or ground flaxseeds*
*1/2 cup bentonite clay*
*2 tablespoons ground psyllium husks or seeds*

*2 tablespoons activated charcoal (optional), or take the tablets*
*2 to 3 tablespoons apple or citrus pectin*

Mix all the ingredients together in a glass jar and refrigerate.

For your fiber shake, combine 1 to 1 1/2 heaping tablespoons of this mixture in 8 ounces of water or fresh vegetable juice and shake well. For added flavor, you can mix in 1 teaspoon of lemon, lime, or unsweetened cranberry juice concentrate.

# Cleansing Herbs and Supplements

There are many commercial colon-cleansing products available that make use of various herbs and nutrients that are beneficial for moving the bowels. You will want to choose a product that works well for you. The goal is to get your bowels moving two to three times a day and to gently and naturally cleanse the walls of the colon to remove impacted material and eliminate stored toxins.

Magnesium is an excellent mineral that helps alleviate constipation by drawing water into the intestines, causing the feces to soften. Herbs that help in colon cleansing include Cape aloe leaf, aloe vera leaf, barberry root, dandelion root, fringe-tree bark, amla fruit, belleric myrobalan fruit, chebulic myrobalan fruit, meadowsweet aerial parts, English plantain aerial parts, fenugreek seeds, licorice root, slippery elm bark, marshmallow root, peppermint leaf, coriander, gentian, cinnamon, rhubarb root, papaya, cayenne, peppermint or spearmint, garlic, fennel seeds, and gingerroot. Cascara sagrada and senna are stimulant herbs with a laxative effect; they can be too harsh for some people. You will not find all these ingredients in every formula, but you should find many of them in a good formula. They can be quite beneficial during a colon cleanse but should not be used in the long term as they can create dependence. Some people are so constipated that they need a formula that includes one or both cascara sagrada and senna, along with more soothing herbs like slippery elm, marshmallow root, and peppermint (see the Resources Guide).

## THE COLON-CLEANSE JUICE COCKTAIL

1 cucumber, washed, or peeled
   if not organic
1 handful spinach, washed
1 handful parsley, washed

1 celery rib, washed
1/2 medium lemon, peeled
1/2 green apple (optional)

Cut the cucumber in half or to the size that will fit your juicer feed tube. Bunch up the spinach and parsley and push them through the juicer with the cucumber, celery, lemon, and apple, if using.

## AWESOME GREEN SMOOTHIE

1 small to medium cucumber,
   washed, or peeled if not
   organic
2 cups spinach, washed
1 medium to large avocado,
   peeled, seed removed

1 tablespoon virgin coconut oil
   (optional)
Juice from 1 lime or lemon
Several drops of stevia to
   sweeten (optional)

Cut the cucumber into chunks, put it in your blender, and process until smooth. Add the spinach and blend until smooth. Cut the avocado into chunks, and add it to the blender along with the coconut oil, if using, lime juice, and stevia, if using. Blend until smooth. Add a little water, as needed. To serve, pour into bowls. If you prefer, you can store the second serving in a container for use later in the day.

SERVES 2

**Note:** This smoothie is good served with chopped or ground raw almonds that have been soaked overnight in the refrigerator for easy digestion and then dehydrated. In fact, all nuts can be digested better if they are first soaked in water, because soaking releases enzyme inhibitors. You can soak and then dehydrate nuts in advance; they taste best prepared this way. To prepare, place them in the dehydrator overnight or until crisp. When you're ready to use them, grind the nuts and sprinkle them on top of the smoothie.

## *Colon Detoxification Helpers*

### PROBIOTICS

As you cleanse, it's very important to restore healthy intestinal flora (bacteria) in the gut by taking what is known as a probiotic (beneficial bacteria) formula. Often, the body's beneficial bacteria have been depleted by the use of antibiotics, other medications, and years of poor eating habits. Probiotics also restore healthful bacteria after cleansing. Proper bacteria are essential for a strong immune system; assimilation of vitamins, minerals, proteins, fats, and carbohydrates; the manufacture of B vitamins; and the control of yeasts such as *Candida albicans* and parasites. (For recommendations, see the Resources Guide.) Depending on the formula you choose as your probiotic, you may need to take probiotics more or less often than is recommended on the menu schedule.

### COLONICS

Colon hydrotherapy, which is popularly known as a colonic, entails flushing the colon with water, usually by a professional colon therapist. Colon hydrotherapy is a safe, effective method of removing waste from the large intestine, without the use of drugs. Intestinal waste is softened and loosened by introducing pure, filtered, temperature-regulated water into the colon, which results in evacuation of waste. A colonic or two per week during the one to two weeks of colon cleansing is particularly beneficial in removing excess waste. It can also be helpful in facilitating weight loss.

If you're thinking, "No way would I consider this," it might be of interest to know that some of the most glamorous people we watch in the media have taken advantage of this health practice. It's been reported that Princess Diana was an avid fan of colonics, and it's rumored that numerous Hollywood stars regularly go for colonics. The reason partakers range from royalty to Hollywood stars to everyday people is that colonics help reduce bloating and gas, flatten protruding tummies, facilitate weight loss, improve colon health, and beautify the skin. I've combined colonics with juice fasting and intestinal herbal cleansing several times a year for more than fifteen years, and on more than one occasion, I've experienced a 2-pound weight loss after a colonic.

Toxins can build up on the intestinal wall just like plaque builds up on teeth. Can you imagine never having your teeth cleaned? Colon irrigation hydrates the colon and assists in the removal of built-up fecal matter, mucus, and toxins.

Although it might be disconcerting to the very shy, most practitioners will immediately make you feel relaxed, at ease, and safe. However, make sure the center you choose is clean and uses disposable hoses and tubes.

People who get colonics usually rave about the effects they experience, such as improved colon health, a flatter stomach, a clearing of the whites of their eyes, improvement in skin health and appearance, and a luminescence to their skin and hair. If you cannot find a colon therapist in your area, enemas are the next best thing.

## THE ENEMA

Enemas have been used for centuries to maintain bowel health. They can be very beneficial in restoring regularity. It was common practice for past generations to use enemas to treat nearly every illness. During a colon cleanse, an enema is excellent for clearing out the debris that is being released from intestinal walls.

An enema entails infusing water into the colon through the anus. You can find enema bags in some drugstores (usually the independent stores, or you may need to order online). The easiest to use are those that look like a hot water bag with a tube. You simply fill the bag with about 1 quart of warm water—filtered or distilled is best—then lie down on your left side, and insert the end of the hose into your anus, making sure the clamp is on tightly so the water doesn't go all over the floor. If you'll remember from our discussion of the anatomy of the colon, the descending colon runs down the left side of the body. This is why it's best to lie down on the left side starting out. Reach behind for the clamp to release it and let the water run in until you start to feel full; then clamp it off for a moment. Unclamp and continue until all the water has drained into your colon. Relax and wait for a few minutes on your left side; then turn on your back for a couple of minutes to allow the water to go across your transverse colon (unless you just can't wait; sometimes, in the beginning, this is hard to do). Next you should turn onto your right side for a couple of minutes so the water can go into the ascending colon. After this you will want to evacuate all the water and waste. Take the time to let everything be expelled. Then relax and stay close to the bathroom for another ten to fifteen minutes.

There are a number of substances that you can add to the water as infusions that can help facilitate the removal of toxic material. Wheatgrass juice is very beneficial because it contains so many healing nutrients and the chlorophyll is detoxifying. It can be made by adding 1 to 2 ounces of wheatgrass juice to 2 cups of warm water. Coffee enemas are sometimes used, and there are people who swear by them. Make sure you use only organic coffee. The simplest and easiest enema is just warm water.

## Exercises to Facilitate Colon Cleansing

The benefits of exercise for overall health and wellness are undisputed. Exercise increases energy, helps you lose weight, increases muscle strength and tone, and helps in cardiovascular fitness. During cleansing, exercise assists in the elimination of toxins. Specific benefits during cleansing include the following:

◆ Increased blood flow so more oxygen reaches your cells and more toxins can be picked up to be eliminated

◆ Decreased stress and anxiety so the entire digestive system can work more efficiently

- Increased lymph flow, which is crucial for the removal of toxins and for increased immune function
- Increased sweating so toxins can be eliminated through the skin
- Increased rate of breathing to eliminate toxins through the lungs

Aerobic exercises are particularly beneficial during cleansing because they increase your heart rate over a sustained time, which boosts oxygen flow through the blood and into every cell in your body. Start with as much as you are able to do. If you aren't accustomed to exercise, work up to at least twenty to thirty minutes or more of sustained movement for maximum benefit at least three days a week; eventually increase to sixty minutes, for a minimum of three times per week. Examples of aerobic exercise include running, jogging, fast walking, swimming, bicycling, dancing, skating, step aerobics classes, or rebounding. Rebounding is one of the best exercises you can do to assist your body during the process of detoxification. It's an exercise performed on a mini trampoline, which is appropriately called a rebounder. It's fun, easy to do, safe, and very effective. You can jump on it in the comfort of your own home—no need to pound the pavement, avoid cars, or put up with bad weather. It's also a zero-impact aerobic exercise that improves blood circulation and increases the capacity of both the heart and the lungs. Moreover, it is one of the most effective exercises for moving the fluids of the lymphatic system, which carry waste products out of our bodies. Vigorous exercise such as rebounding can significantly increase lymph flow. Because lymph is totally dependent on physical exercise (or lymphatic drainage massage) to move, without adequate movement the lymph system cannot properly excrete toxic waste products, which in turn affects the cells, limiting their ability to efficiently absorb life-giving nutrients.

Exercise is very important for the lymphatic system because there is no active lymph pump to move lymph through the lymph vessels like the heart pumps blood through the blood vessels. The lymphatic system is passive, not active, and the vessels of the lymphatic system have valves that move it in one direction only. Therefore, active movement is required to keep the fluids moving. The main lymph vessels run up the legs, arms, and torso, so an up-and-down movement is especially effective at pumping lymph through the vessels. An excellent machine to move lymph through the body and to exercise the internal organs is known as the lymphasizer, or swing machine. It's a small unit with a remote control that has grooves for your ankles. You lie on the floor with your feet in the grooves and the machine does the rest. I've experienced firsthand how effective this machine is at moving lymph. (See the Resources Guide.)

Regardless of what activity you do, the main point during a cleanse is to exert yourself enough to increase your rate of breathing and break a sweat. The process of sweating greatly facilitates the removal of toxins, which will make your detoxing much easier and more effective. In addition to exercise, saunas, either infrared or regular, and hot soaking baths, especially in natural mineral springs, will induce sweating and facilitate the elimination of toxins.

### Intestinal Cleansing for Vibrant Health: Summary

**Step 1:**  Eat whole, alkalizing foods, emphasizing organic, non-GMO foods. Remove as many sources of toxicity as possible, drink plenty of water, and eat 50 to 75 percent of your food raw.

**Step 2:**  Add fresh vegetable juices to your diet at least once or twice a day.

**Step 3:**  Complete one to three days of juice fasting.

**Step 4:**  Perform the colon detoxification program

- Increase your consumption of water, juice, and herbal tea to flush out toxins.
- Eat colon-cleansing foods and limit colon-clogging foods (see box on pages 129–30).
- Add a fiber shake four times during the day.
- Take an herbal cleansing formula one or more times daily (follow product directions).
- Take a colonic or an enema at least once or twice during the program.
- Add aerobic exercises to increase your heart rate and induce sweating.
- Take saunas or hot baths during the cleanse to facilitate sweating.

# CHAPTER SIX

## *Liver, Gallbladder, and Kidney Cleansing*

If your washing machine was broken down, your drain was clogged, or your water heater was leaking, you'd get to work right away to make repairs. Your liver, gallbladder, and kidneys are far more important than any household appliance, yet they often get far less attention. Isn't it time to cleanse these hardworking organs and get them in good working condition again?

The detox programs that follow will help you cleanse the liver, gallbladder, and kidneys and assist them in functioning well so you can feel healthy, energetic, and really alive. It may seem strange to think that the liver, gallbladder, and kidneys have something to do with how you feel, but they do. Their health is key to your overall health. You'll never know just how good you can feel until you cleanse these organs of elimination. So let's get started with the liver detoxification program.

## Liver Detoxification

The liver is the largest and most complex internal organ in the human body. It performs hundreds of tasks every minute of every day, more than any other organ, including the brain. The brain processes information like a computer, but the liver processes physiological tasks like a busy work crew. It's constantly filtering, detoxifying, synthesizing, and processing a wide variety of substances. Without a healthy, well-functioning liver, you can quickly become toxic, which leads to feeling tired, sick, and often depressed. You might notice your fingers and toes aren't as thin as they once were, because impaired liver function causes decreased serum albumen, which leads to edema, or swelling due to fluid accumulation in the tissues. Or maybe your hormones are out of whack because the liver metabolizes most hormones, and when it's not functioning well, hormone metabolism is off.

The liver is the main organ of detoxification in the body, filtering and cleansing approximately fifty gallons of blood every day. The liver acts much like a coffee filter in straining out harmful toxins and ammonia. They're removed from the blood and transformed before being eliminated through the bowels or the kidneys. The liver also processes the pollutants that we breathe in through our lungs or absorb through our skin. Whether toxins are from environmental pollution or processed or contaminated food or are internally produced, they're all detoxified in the liver in a complex, two-step process known as phase 1 and phase 2 detoxification. Each of these phases requires specific nutrients to perform the work properly. In this program, the nutrients are supplied by juices, raw soups, green smoothies, whole organic foods, and nutritional supplements. These foods support the liver and enable it to break down the toxic and congestive stuff we don't want and move it from one phase to the next. Without adequate nutrients, and especially antioxidants, detoxification can stall, which allows the free radicals that are formed during the intermediate process to proliferate, causing more damaged cells and further problems. But with plenty of nutrients, fat-soluble toxins that would otherwise be stored in fat cells and cell membranes can be converted into water-soluble forms that are subsequently excreted through the kidneys or via the bile that dumps into the colon.

In addition to detoxification, the liver performs numerous other tasks that are crucial to life and health. Many of these functions directly affect energy production, so when the liver is congested, its ability to produce energy is reduced. The main energy-producing functions include the following:

- Regulating carbohydrate metabolism, which controls blood sugar
- Regulating protein metabolism, which produces proteins that transport substances such as fat and hormones
- Burning fat for fuel, as well as making cholesterol and fat and storing it
- Regulating hormonal metabolism, especially converting T4 to T3 (thyroid hormones); T4 goes mostly to the liver, where it is converted to T3

The liver holds a key to efficient metabolism, weight control, bowel health, and detoxification. Good function is especially crucial for weight loss, in that the liver is the major fat-burning organ in the body. Cleansing your liver can greatly improve your ability to lose weight and increase your energy so you feel more like exercising.

When you regularly consume sweets and other processed carbohydrates (like bread, rolls, pizza, and pasta), junk food, artificial sweeteners, and beverages such as soft drinks and alcohol, your liver converts most of these calories to fat and stores it, and you gain weight. Did you know that sugar and foods that easily convert to sugar are major contributors to high cholesterol? High blood sugar contributes to higher LDL cholesterol and lower HDL cholesterol. High blood sugar also damages the lining of your arteries.

Because of the increased use of high fructose corn syrup in soft drinks, fruit juices, salad dressings, condiments, and processed foods, fat can build up in the liver. This is becoming more common than it ever has been, which can lead to "fatty liver." When this happens, something has gone wrong with the metabolism. It's known that fat accumulates in the liver with a number of conditions—the most common being obesity, and it is also associated with insulin resistance, metabolic syndrome, type 2 diabetes, high triglycerides, and heavy use of alcohol. For all these reasons, you want to get the sugars and especially high fructose corn syrup, refined carbs, processed foods, and junk out of your diet.

The liver stores toxins in its cells. The more toxins it stores, the more the liver functions are compromised. The liver can become congested just like the colon. It can also develop stones. When the liver is congested, excretion of bile is slowed down, and you'll be more prone to constipation. This leads to toxins lingering in the gut too long, and some will be absorbed back into the bloodstream. Toxins circulating in the system can cause water retention in certain areas of the body, especially the thighs, hips, and arms, because the body holds on to the extra water to dilute toxins. This leads to cellulite—that unsightly, bumpy skin. A cleansed, well-functioning liver can greatly facilitate the loss of cellulite and water weight.

### Liver Toxicity, Weight Gain, and High Cholesterol

The liver can push fat out of the body through the bile into the small intestines. It is a remarkable organ when it comes to keeping weight under control, since it's both a fat-burning and a fat-pumping organ. When it stops burning fat because of congestion, it will become a fat-storing organ. That's when people stop losing weight or can't even begin their weight-loss journey, no matter how much they starve themselves. When the liver doesn't regulate fat metabolism efficiently, weight gain tends to occur around the midsection and a protruding belly can develop. Some people acquire a roll of fat around the abdomen. It can be nearly impossible to lose abdominal fat until liver function is improved. Once this is done, the liver will start burning fat efficiently again and the weight comes off gradually and without a lot of effort.

A high-fiber diet will reduce the recirculation of fat and toxins from the gut back to the liver. This is important for those with excessive weight, toxicity, or high cholesterol. The inclusion of plenty of raw fruits and vegetables as well as raw seeds will increase both soluble and insoluble fiber in the gut and reduce recirculation of unwanted fat and toxins. You may also find apple pectin and psyllium husks beneficial to boost fiber intake.

If the liver is damaged by toxins or clogged with excessive waste, it will be less efficient at removing small fat globules circulating in the blood. This will cause excessive fat to build up on blood vessel walls.

It can also build up in many other parts of the body, including the liver and other organs, and in fatty deposits under the skin. You may develop cellulite in the buttocks, thighs, arms, and abdomen. If the liver is dysfunctional, it will not manufacture adequate amounts of HDL, which scavenges the unhealthy LDL from the blood vessel walls.

If the liver's filtering system is healthy, it allows dietary cholesterol to be shunted into the liver for metabolism or excretion through the bile. A healthy liver is essential to properly regulate cholesterol levels. High cholesterol can be a sign of a fatty or toxic liver. Poor liver function may increase your chances of cardiovascular diseases such as atherosclerosis, high blood pressure, heart attacks, and strokes.

You may have a number of signs of liver congestion, even though all your liver-function blood tests appear normal. The tests used to determine liver function are not designed to show mild dysfunction, but rather liver damage. Because the liver is involved in so many critical functions, it can affect nearly every system in your body, including the nervous system, immune system, endocrine system, digestive system, and circulatory system. So if you have even a couple of the symptoms listed below, it's a great idea to get going on a liver cleanse.

### Symptoms of Liver Dysfunction

- Acne, allergies, or asthma
- Allergic conditions such as hay fever, hives, skin rashes, asthma
- Back pain
- Brown or dark spots on the skin, often called age spots or liver spots
- Bursitis
- Cancer
- Candidiasis
- Coated tongue or bad breath in the morning
- Fatigue or chronic fatigue syndrome
- Fluid retention: swollen legs, fingers, or toes
- Headaches: migraines, tension headaches, hormonal headaches, cluster headaches, pain in the eyes, vision problems

*(Continued)*

- High blood pressure
- Hypoglycemia or blood sugar instability
- Immune system weakness
- Inability to tolerate fatty foods
- Insomnia
- Irritable bowel syndrome
- Kidney problems
- Lupus
- Mood changes, depression, or "foggy" brain
- Nausea or abdominal pains
- Acid reflux
- Obesity
- Poor digestion, bloating, gas, weight gain, cellulite, or constipation
- Sinus problems
- Small bright red spots on the body (called cherry angiomas)
- Thin stools (diameter of a rope or pencil)

When you detoxify your liver, it should give a big sigh of relief and go on about its job of detoxifying, regulating metabolism, and burning fat. When the liver is working well, you'll feel and look better. Weight loss should be easy and natural, without excessive effort, and your immune system should function more efficiently, making it easier to stay healthy all year.

## Gallbladder Detoxification

The liver and gallbladder are interconnected and work together. What affects one affects the other—both positively and negatively. One of the primary routes of eliminating toxins is through the bile, which is made in the liver and concentrated and stored in the gallbladder. Bile helps break down fats and fat-soluble vitamins when it's secreted into the small intestine. Its other main function is to transport toxins from the liver. It's somewhat like a garbage truck, picking up toxic waste from the liver and transporting it down the bile duct "highway" into the bowels to be excreted through the colon.

Bile contains water, cholesterol, fat, bile salts, proteins, and bilirubin. If it contains too much cholesterol, bile salts, or bilirubin, due principally to inefficient liver function, it can sometimes harden into pieces of stonelike material called gallstones. There are two types of gallstones: cholesterol stones and pigment stones. Cholesterol stones are made from hardened cholesterol and are a yellow-green color. They account for about 80 percent of all gallstones. Pigment stones, which are small, dark stones, are made up principally of bilirubin. The gallbladder can develop stones of all sizes, from hundreds of tiny stones to one large stone. If a stone gets stuck in the duct that carries bile from the liver to the small intestine, it can block the flow of bile, which causes inflammation and pain. In addition to forming from too much cholesterol (often related to a diet high in animal products) or too much bilirubin, stones can form from a deficiency of bile salts or because the gallbladder is not efficient enough to properly secrete bile.

Intense pain in the abdomen that radiates to the upper back or upper right shoulder can be an indication of gallstones. Ultrasound provides a definitive diagnosis. Approximately 20 percent of women and 8 percent of men over forty in the United States experience gallstones. Each year this leads to surgery to remove more than three hundred thousand gallbladders. It's far better to periodically complete a liver/gallbladder detox than to undergo the pain and expense of gallbladder surgery, which can adversely affect your health thereafter. After all, your body was meant to have a gallbladder.

## SYMPTOMS OF GALLBLADDER PROBLEMS

People can have digestive problems for years, and because these problems are interrelated with other digestive symptoms, they may never realize that their problems may be related to the gallbladder. Constipation is one of the most commonly missed symptoms of gallbladder problems. The following list refers to symptoms associated with gallbladder problems, but keep in mind they could also be indicative of something else. One thing is certain: It's better to cleanse and support your gallbladder at the first sign of problems or before any problems show up than to lose it.

- Pain or tenderness under the rib cage on the right side
- Pain between the shoulder blades
- Pain around the right shoulder blade
- Light or chalky-colored stools
- Indigestion after eating, especially after eating fatty or greasy foods
- Nausea
- Dizziness
- Bloating
- Gas
- Burping or belching
- Feeling of fullness or poor food digestion
- Diarrhea (or alternating from soft to watery stools)

- Constipation
- Headache over the eyes, especially the right eye
- Bitter fluid reflux after eating
- Frequent need for laxatives

### Diet for a Happy Liver and Gallbladder

There are certain foods, beverages, and lifestyle choices that can lead to health and wellness for the liver/gallbladder team. We call these liver-friendly foods and lifestyle choices. Those choices that undermine or interfere with this team's wellness are called liver-unfriendly.

**LIVER-FRIENDLY**

- Organic vegetables and vegetable juices
- Organic fruit
- Organic raw nuts and seeds
- Organic legumes
- Organic whole grains
- Free-range poultry and grass-fed meats
- Fish (wild-caught)
- Organic free-range eggs
- Good fats and oils (extra-virgin olive oil, coconut oil, fish oil)
- Plenty of filtered or distilled water
- Herb tea, green tea, or white tea
- Exercise, especially aerobic
- Positive, life-affirming attitudes, thoughts, and words
- Moderate eating
- Adequate sleep

**LIVER-UNFRIENDLY**

- Refined, processed, and canned foods
- Sweet foods, treats, and desserts
- Fast foods (e.g., French fries, burgers, pizza, and tacos)
- Deep-fried foods
- Refined flour products (bread, pasta, pizza dough, and bagels)
- Fatty meats, preserved meats, and cold cuts
- Hydrogenated and partially hydrogenated fats (margarine)
- Trans fats and polyunsaturated vegetable oils such as soy, corn, canola, sunflower, and safflower
- Alcohol, coffee, and soft drinks
- Sedentary lifestyle
- Stress, anxiety, anger, worry, and fear
- Negative attitudes, thoughts, and words
- Overeating

# My First Experience with Gallbladder Cleansing

When I had chronic fatigue syndrome and fibromyalgia and I was so sick I couldn't work, I sought help wherever I could find it. One of the people I contacted was a reflexologist. I called him the Mountain Man of Colorado. Reflexology is the application of pressure to specific points and areas on the feet, hands, or ears—most often it's the feet. Reflexologists believe that these areas and reflex points correspond to different body organs and systems and that pressing the points has a beneficial effect on the organs and a person's overall health. For example, reflexology states that a specific spot in the arch of the foot corresponds to the liver/gallbladder point. When my reflexologist pressed on the liver/gallbladder point, I about flew out of my chair—it hurt that much. He said it was obvious that I needed to do a gallbladder flush. His recommendation was 1 cup of freshly made apple juice and 1 cup of extra-virgin olive oil, warmed, and placed in a jar to shake vigorously until it was well blended. Drinking that was fierce. And at six a.m., it was even worse. It was about the nastiest thing I've ever tasted. Then I was to go back to bed for a couple of hours and lie on my right side. This was to flush out stones. I slept more than two hours. When I got up, I was quite disappointed because nothing happened—no stones eliminated. I kept thinking, "How disappointing that I went through all that for nothing." But around four p.m., I thought I was going to die, with a lot of pain in my abdomen.

That's when my body expelled what seemed to be a couple of hundred stones of varying sizes and colors. I was totally amazed.

What I did is not what I would recommend for you. A stone could get stuck and send you to the emergency room. The programs that follow are gentle and gradually help soften stones and prepare your body for a flush, if you choose to do one.

## The Seven-Day Liver/Gallbladder Detoxification Program

A thorough detoxification program is best done at least twice a year, around the spring and the fall. For optimum health you may want to cleanse four times a year, once at each change of season.

An effective liver/gallbladder detoxification program includes these six important steps:

1. Reduce your exposure to toxins—from the environment and from processed, preserved foods.
2. Avoid coffee, alcohol, tobacco, junk food, all sweets, refined grains (wheat, rye, barley), soft drinks, and over-the-counter medications.
3. Eat a health-building, whole, organic foods diet—with plenty of raw vegetables, fruit, and fresh vegetable juices.
4. Exercise—sweat to eliminate toxins (saunas are also very helpful).

5. Drink plenty of water to flush toxins (2 to 2 1/2 quarts a day).

6. Use detoxification programs designed for your liver and gallbladder (see pages 172–78).

For seven days, you will follow this menu plan and utilize vegetable juice and green smoothie recipes in this book or your own favorites, adding plenty of fresh raw vegetables and a small amount of low-sugar fruit as desired. During this cleanse you will not be eating any animal products, but you can have as many fresh raw vegetables, green smoothies, vegetable juices, and steamed or sautéed vegetables as you wish, so you should not experience hunger.

Choose plenty of leafy green vegetables such as lettuce, spinach, Swiss chard, parsley, and mustard greens, as well as cruciferous vegetables such as broccoli, cauliflower, cabbage, Brussels sprouts, and kale. Greens are rich in essential vitamins, minerals, enzymes, phytonutrients, antioxidants, biophotons, and chlorophyll. They help your body detoxify and reach an alkaline pH, which is especially needed during a detox program.

You may want to supplement your diet with a concentrated, powdered greens formula that contains organically grown grasses such as wheatgrass, barley grass, and oat grass. Many products also contain spirulina, sprouted grains, herbs, and green vegetables. The concentrated greens can help in the detoxification process (see the Resources Guide).

## Liver/Gallbladder-Friendly Vegetables

Eat an abundance of the following liver/gallbladder-friendly vegetables during the seven days of your detoxification program:

- Artichokes
- Beets
- Broccoli
- Brussels sprouts
- Cabbage
- Carrots
- Cauliflower
- Celery
- Chives
- Cucumber
- Eggplant
- Garlic
- Green beans
- Jerusalem artichokes (sun chokes)
- Kale
- Kohlrabi
- Lettuce
- Mustard greens
- Okra
- Onions
- Parsley
- Parsnips
- Peas
- Pumpkin
- Spinach
- Squash
- Sweet potatoes or yams

There are two menu plans that you may choose from. Both of these plans are very effective for cleansing the liver and gallbladder. Option 1 involves a little more preparation, but less expense. It's for people who have the time to prepare special juices and salads, along with a few recommended herbs, but who do not want to spend much extra money on special liver/gallbladder-cleansing herbs and teas. Option 2 is similar in many ways but involves less time in preparation and entails purchasing cleansing herbs and teas. Choose from either option and follow as outlined for the full seven days.

The best time to do this seven-day program, if you work outside the home or go to school, is to start on the weekend, when you have a little more time to get personal things done.

Then you can prepare the juices, green smoothies, and salads ahead of time for the rest of the detox days and take what you need to work in a cooler for the remaining days. (You can freeze the juices.) Option 2 is usually easier for people who work away from home, but you will still need to prepare mostly raw foods and juices to take with you.

In addition to following the menu options, keep in mind the importance of a cleansed colon that moves freely. If you become constipated or your bowels are not moving every day, add fiber supplements and herbs (see chapter five, "Intestinal Cleansing for Vibrant Health").

## MENU PLAN FOR OPTION 1

**Upon Rising**

**7:00 A.M. or upon rising** Drink 1 cup purified water.

**7:15 A.M.** Drink the Blended Citrus Shake.

### BLENDED CITRUS SHAKE

You will consume this shake every morning.

*1 cup distilled or purified water*
*Juice of 1 lemon and 1 lime*
*1-inch piece fresh gingerroot, cut into pieces*
*1 to 5 cloves garlic (On day 1 use 1 garlic clove; on day 2 use 2 garlic cloves; continue adding one garlic*
*clove per day until day 5, when you'll use 5 garlic cloves.)*
*1 to 5 tablespoons extra-virgin, cold-pressed olive oil (On day 1 use 1 tablespoon; on day 2 use 2 tablespoons; continue adding 1 tablespoon per*

*day until day 5, when
you'll use 5 tablespoons. If
you want do the complete
gallbladder flush, then
on days 6 and 7 you use
5 garlic cloves and 5*

*tablespoons of olive oil.)*
*1 tablespoon virgin coconut oil
(optional)*
*2 to 4 ice cubes, made with
filtered or distilled water
(optional)*

Place all ingredients in a blender and blend at high speed for about 1 minute or until ingredients are well combined. Pour into a large glass and drink it all. This shake will stimulate your liver and begin to flush out toxins.

## Breakfast

### 8:00–9:00 A.M.

- Have the Beet-Cucumber Cleansing Cocktail (page 298); if desired, you can add the juice to a blender with an avocado; blend until smooth to make a smoothie.
- Eat 1 to 2 teaspoons Beet Salad (page 181); beets are fabulous for liver detoxification and support, so you'll be consuming beet salad throughout the day.
- Take a supplement: 1 to 2 capsules of the herb milk thistle or liver-cleansing herbs or tincture (see the Resources Guide).

**10:00 A.M.** Drink the Gallbladder-Cleansing Cocktail (page 183).

**10:30 A.M.** Drink 8 ounces purified water.

**11:00 A.M.** Eat 1 to 2 teaspoons Beet Salad.

**11:30 A.M.** Drink ginger or echinacea herbal tea, or a commercial detoxification tea.

## Lunch

### 12:00 Noon

- Choose any smoothie or raw soup recipe from the recipe section.
- If you're still hungry, add a vegetable salad or raw vegetable sticks.
- Take a supplement: 1 to 2 capsules of the herb milk thistle or liver-cleansing herbs.

**1:15 P.M.** Eat 1 to 2 teaspoons Beet Salad.

**2:00 P.M.** Drink 8 ounces purified water or herbal tea.

**3:00 P.M.**

- Have a Green Drink (page 182): Juice as many greens as you like. Start with a base of cucumber, celery, and lemon. To that add parsley, kale, spinach, sprouts, or any other greens. If juice is not possible, mix powdered greens in water.
- Eat 1 to 2 teaspoons Beet Salad.

**4:30 P.M.**

- Drink 8 ounces purified water.
- Eat 1 to 2 teaspoons Beet Salad.

## Dinner

**5:00 P.M.** Drink 8 ounces purified water.

**6:00 P.M.**

- Eat the Carrot Salad with Lemon–Olive Oil Dressing (page 181).
- Drink 1 cup Potassium-Rich Vegetable Broth (page 182).

- Have a vegetable salad or blended vegetable soup. You may substitute cooked artichokes, which are very liver supportive, but no dressing or dip other than olive oil and lemon juice.
- Take a supplement: 1 to 2 capsules milk thistle or liver-cleansing herbs.

**7:15 P.M.** Eat 1 to 2 teaspoons Beet Salad.

**8:30 P.M.** Drink chamomile or peppermint herbal tea.

**Make sure you consume at least 64 ounces (eight 8-ounce glasses) of water per day.**

## MENU PLAN FOR OPTION 2

For recommendations of products that can work well with this program, see the Resources Guide.

### Upon Rising

**7:00 A.M. or upon rising** Drink 1 cup distilled or filtered water (distilled is best for detoxing).

**7:15 A.M.** Drink the Blended Citrus Shake (page 172).

**7:30 A.M.** Drink 2 cups detoxification tea and/or liver/gallbladder herbal formulas according to manufacturer's directions (see the Resources Guide).

### Breakfast

**8:30 A.M.** Alternate between these two choices (optional: add a concentrated greens powder to either choice; see the Resources Guide):

I.  Beet-Cucumber Cleansing Cocktail (page 298); if
    desired, you can then add the juice to a blender with
    an avocado; blend until smooth.

2.  Gallbladder-Cleansing Cocktail (page 183).

## Midmorning

- Drink 2 cups commercial detoxification tea (see the
  Resources Guide).
- Take liver/gallbladder herbal formulas; follow
  manufacturer's directions (see the Resources Guide).

## Lunch

### 12:00 Noon

- **Days 1 and 5:** You may have a vegetable salad, raw
  vegetable sticks, or lightly steamed vegetables such
  as broccoli or cooked artichoke. Or choose from
  any of the juice, smoothie, or raw soup recipes. For
  salad dressing, choose from olive oil, lemon juice,
  avocado, garlic, Bragg Liquid Aminos, or any spices
  or herbs. (You can combine all these ingredients or
  some of them, as desired.)
- **Days 2 through 4:** Choose any juice, smoothie, or
  raw soup recipe from the recipe section. You will
  not be consuming any solid food on these days,
  which are a three-day juice fast.

## Midafternoon

- Drink 2 cups detoxification tea.

- Take liver/gallbladder herbal formulas according to the manufacturer's directions (see the Resources Guide).

**Dinner**

**6:00 P.M.**

- **Days 1 and 5:** You may have a vegetable salad, raw vegetable sticks, lightly steamed vegetables such as broccoli or cooked artichoke, raw food dishes, dehydrated veggies, and dehydrated crackers. Or choose from any of the juice, smoothie, or raw soup recipes. For salad dressing, choose from olive oil, lemon juice, avocado, garlic, Bragg Liquid Aminos, or any spices or herbs. (Combine all these ingredients or just the ones you desire.)
- **Days 2 through 4:** Choose any juice, smoothie, or raw soup recipe from the recipe section, or have 1 cup Potassium-Rich Vegetable Broth (page 182). You will not be consuming any solid food on these days. You will break the juice fast on day 4 with a raw soup and a dehydrated cracker, as desired. On day 5 you will have solid foods and juices and smoothies.

**Evening**

Drink herb teas of your choice.

**Liver/Gallbladder Detoxification Programs: Summary**

- Increase consumption of water, vegetable juice, and herb teas to flush toxins.
- Follow detoxification menu plan, either Option 1 or Option 2.
- Drink Blended Citrus Shake every morning.
- Eat liver-friendly foods and eliminate liver-unfriendly foods (see box, page 167).
- Eat no animal foods during this cleanse.
- Take herbal liver-cleanse formulas and drink detoxing teas (use according to manufacturer's directions) if following Option 2.
- Add aerobic exercises to increase heart rate and cause sweating.
- Take saunas or hot baths to facilitate sweating.

When you have finished your liver/gallbladder cleanse, eat only whole foods and follow the basic cleansing steps until you are ready to go on to either the kidney flush or a second liver/gallbladder cleanse that includes an optional sixth day of intensive gallbladder cleansing (see "Why Complete an Intensive Gallbladder Flush?").

# Why Complete an Intensive Gallbladder Flush?

You may be one of the millions of people who have one or many gallstones that have accumulated in the gallbladder or liver. These stones or material can be in the form of little rocks, sand, or muddy substances. If you suspect you have gallstones, or are over forty and have eaten a typical American diet, or have never done a liver or gallbladder cleanse and just want to be sure your gallbladder is as clean as possible, you may want to try the intensive gallbladder flush.

Before you do this flush, you will need to complete five days of the liver/gallbladder detoxification program as outlined on pages 169–172. This program will help soften stones and increase bile solubility. The intensive gallbladder flush will aggressively go after stubborn stones that may still be in your gallbladder or liver.

On your liver/gallbladder detox, plan a day, such as a Saturday, when you have some time to devote yourself to the cleanse. On the evening of the sixth day, follow the intensive gallbladder flush exactly as outlined below. On the seventh day you may pass stones of various sizes and colors.

> **Note:** If you try the intensive gallbladder flush prematurely, the gallbladder could release a large stone that could block the bile duct, which would require immediate surgery. Before embarking on the intensive sixth-day gallbladder flush, you may wish to consult your health care professional.

If you have problems with constipation or a sluggish colon, you could benefit by using the colon-cleansing Homemade Fiber Blend formulas (see pages 147–48) or a premade colon-cleanse formula (see the Resources Guide) during your liver/gallbladder detoxification program. You may want to take an enema as outlined in chapter five (pages 153–54) to be sure your colon is moving efficiently before you begin the intensive sixth-day gallbladder flush. Make sure you eat no animal products during this flush.

## *The Intensive Sixth-Day Gallbladder Flush*

> **Note:** Do this only after you have completed five days of the liver/gallbladder detox program. The intensive gallbladder flush is done on the sixth day of your liver/gallbladder detoxification program. I no longer recommend using Epsom salts since they are hard on your organs of elimination.

Choose a day like Saturday for the intensive flush, when you can rest most of the day.

- Take no medications (except mandatory prescription medication) or nutritional supplements on this day.
- Drink only fresh vegetable juices for breakfast and lunch.
- Eat no solid food on this day.
- **After 2:00 p.m.** Do not drink juices, but drink plenty of water, to which you can add lemon.
- **9:45 p.m.** Pour 1/2 cup extra-virgin olive oil into a saucepan and add 1/2 cup apple juice or grapefruit juice; gently warm over low heat. Pour the mixture into a jar and shake, or pour into a blender and process. Mix thoroughly and drink within 5 minutes. You may want to rinse your mouth afterward.
- **10:00 p.m. or sooner** Lie down in bed on your right side immediately after drinking this mixture. Try to lie still for at least 20 minutes; hopefully, you can go to sleep.
- The next morning, upon awakening, drink 1 cup hot water with lemon.
- One hour later, you may have fresh vegetable juice.
- You may have a fresh garden salad for lunch or a green smoothie or raw soup.

## WHAT SHOULD I EXPECT?

Though this cleanse mixture does not offer an appealing taste, it's worth it because it works. Here's what you can expect:

You may experience diarrhea. Sometime during the morning to afternoon of the seventh day, you should pass gallstones, sand, or mud. Gallstones are usually green and pea-size but can range in size from that of lemon seeds to dimes, and they float. Sand or mud looks about like it sounds. Colors of stones can range from tan, black, and light to dark green to turquoise. I mention this only so you won't be too alarmed by what you see. The upside of what to expect is greatly improved digestion.

## LIVER AND GALLBLADDER DETOX RECIPES AND PRODUCTS

### BEET SALAD

Eat 1 to 2 teaspoons of this salad every 2 to 3 hours during the day for 5 days. You may get tired of eating beets all day, but remember how great it is for your liver. Eating a few teaspoons of this salad every couple of hours is a small price to pay to help your precious liver cleanse and rejuvenate. Don't be alarmed if your stools or urine is red from the beets.

*2 tablespoons extra-virgin, cold-pressed olive oil*
*Juice of 1/2 lemon*
*1 cup finely grated or very finely chopped raw beets (or use the pulp from your juicer after making beet juice)*

*Dash of cinnamon (optional)*
*Whisk the olive oil and lemon juice together and mix with the beets. Add a dash of cinnamon, if desired.*

### CARROT SALAD WITH LEMON–OLIVE OIL DRESSING

*1 cup finely shredded carrots (or carrot pulp left over from juicing)*
*1 tablespoon extra-virgin, cold-pressed olive oil*

*1 tablespoon lemon juice*
*Dash of cinnamon (optional)*

If you are shredding the carrots, they should be a mushy consistency; use a food processor or fine grater. (It's easiest to use carrot pulp.) Place the carrots in a bowl. For the dressing, combine the olive oil with the lemon juice and a dash of cinnamon, if desired. Whisk together. You may add more dressing, but not less. Pour the dressing over the carrots and mix well.

## GREEN DRINK

Preferably in the afternoon, drink 10 ounces of freshly juiced green vegetables—cucumber, parsley, spinach, kale, chard, collards, celery, or any other green herb or vegetable. Add fresh lemon juice and/or freshly juiced gingerroot to pep up the flavor. Fresh mint also makes a nice addition to cucumber and other milder-tasting greens.

## POTASSIUM-RICH VEGETABLE BROTH

This vegetable broth provides important nutrients, especially minerals, your body needs during the cleansing process. Eat 1 to 2 cups of broth daily.

*2 to 3 cups chopped fresh green beans (string beans) (frozen is acceptable when fresh is unavailable)*
*2 to 3 cups chopped zucchini*
*2 to 3 celery ribs*

*Purified water, for steaming*
*1 to 3 tablespoons chopped parsley*
*1 tablespoon chopped garlic*
*Seasonings and herbs, to taste*
*Coconut oil (optional)*

Steam the green beans, zucchini, and celery over purified water until soft, but still green and not mushy. Place the cooked vegetables, plus the parsley and garlic, in a blender and puree until smooth. Add a bit of the steaming water, as needed, but keep the broth fairly thick. Season to taste with minced ginger, cayenne, vegetable seasoning, or herbs of your choice. Add coconut oil, if desired.

SERVES 6 (You can store the extra servings in a jar for later use.)

## GALLBLADDER-CLEANSING COCKTAIL

*1 handful parsley*
*4 medium carrots, scrubbed*
    *well, green tops removed,*
    *ends trimmed*

*2 celery ribs with leaves,*
    *washed, ends trimmed*
*1/2 lemon, peeled*

Bunch up the parsley and push it through the juicer feed tube with the carrots, celery, and lemon. Stir the juice and pour into a glass. If you want a more substantial drink, you can pour the juice into a blender and add an avocado. Blend and serve in a glass or bowl, or you can make it thick like a soup and eat with a spoon by adding more avocado and/or less juice. Drink as soon as possible to maximize the nutritional value; store in the refrigerator, covered; or take with you in a thermos.

SERVES 1

## RECOMMENDATIONS FOR ADDITIONAL FRESH VEGETABLE JUICE

- Carrot, beet, and cucumber juice
- Carrot, celery, and endive or kale juice
- Carrot, beet, and coconut milk
- Carrot and spinach juice

**Note:** If you are sugar sensitive (hypoglycemic or diabetic) and react to carrots or beets, then use cucumber and more greens to dilute your juice, and flavor with lemon juice and ginger. You can also add avocado to the juice and blend until smooth.

## Milk Thistle (Silymarin)

Take one or two capsules of the herb milk thistle with each meal. Milk thistle contains potent liver-cleansing compounds. Silymarin, the most active ingredient in milk thistle, enhances liver function. It also has excellent antioxidant properties that help prevent damage to the liver. Alternatively, you can use a liver-cleansing herbal combination that contains milk thistle.

## Liver/Gallbladder-Cleansing Herbs

There are various cleansing herbal formulas for detoxifying the liver and gallbladder, improving liver function, increasing bile flow, reducing swelling, and purifying the blood. They can be partnered with herbs used to strengthen the liver's glandular and organ functions. Such herbs help remove fat deposits associated with consuming too many unhealthy foods, damaged fats, sugar, and alcohol, as well as chemical exposure. For more information, see the Resources Guide.

## Liver/Gallbladder-Cleansing, -Stimulating, and -Protecting Herbs

It's not recommended that you formulate your own combinations of these herbs, since they are not combined in equal amounts, but rather look for liver/gallbladder-cleansing products that contain some or all of these (see the Resources Guide).

- Artichoke leaf
- Barberry root bark
- Black walnut hull
- Burdock root

- Cardamom seed
- Cinnamon bark
- Clove
- Curcumin
- Dandelion root
- Fennel seed
- Garlic
- Gentian root
- Gingerroot
- Goldenseal root
- Horsetail herb
- Juniper berry

- Licorice root
- Mandrake root
- Milk thistle
- Oregon grape root
- Parsley root
- Pau d'arco bark
- Schisandra
- Turmeric
- Uva-ursi leaf
- Wormwood
- Yellow dock root

**Lipotropic Formula**

A lipotropic formula (which is great for the gallbladder) includes choline, methionine, taurine, betaine hydrochloride, folic acid, and vitamin B6. This combination of nutrients helps remove fat from the liver and increases bile solubility. Take as directed (see the Resources Guide).

---

### The Liver and Emotions

The liver is a doorway into our emotional library. Unexpressed, over-expressed, or denied emotions have the ability to shut down important liver functions. Watch for emotions that surface when you are working on the liver; anger is a typical emotion to pop up. More than any other organ, the liver is affected by negative thoughts, emotions, and feelings. Anger, hate, rage, fear, jealousy, resentment, depression, self-pity, self-unforgiveness, self-rejection, self-bitterness, and hopelessness have a powerfully detrimental impact on the liver.

## Kidney Cleansing

When we cleanse, it's important to include the kidneys, as they are one of the five primary organs for eliminating toxins from the body. The kidneys filter the blood, returning most of the water and many of the dissolved substances back into the bloodstream. What's left is called the urine, which passes through the ureters to the bladder for storage, and finally through the urethra for elimination. Toxins and metabolic waste are eliminated through the urine.

The kidneys have many other important functions, such as the regulation of blood volume and blood pressure, the regulation of ion levels in the blood, and the regulation of blood pH, so it's crucial that they function at peak efficiency.

During cleansing, the kidneys must process more toxic substances than normal, including proteins, salts, and chemicals. If they are congested, we can experience mild symptoms such as water retention or more severe symptoms such as inflammation of kidney tissue. Concentrated protein wastes can result in inflammation of the kidney's filtering tissues (nephritis), causing the bloodstream to become overloaded with toxins. It's also well known that the emotions of fear and insecurity can cause kidney imbalances. In addition, certain prescription drugs can damage the kidneys.

A number of herbs are beneficial in strengthening and toning the kidneys. They help increase urine flow, reduce inflammation, and remove uric acid and other crystalline formations. The five-day kidney flush contains natural foods and herbs that support and cleanse the kidneys.

## SYMPTOMS SIGNALING THAT YOU MAY NEED A KIDNEY CLEANSE

- Changes in urine
- Pain or discomfort near the kidneys
- Pain when urinating
- High blood pressure and swelling
- Anemia
- Muscle cramps
- Contraction of the calf muscles in the leg
- Itching
- Dark circles under the eyes
- Skin rashes
- Loss of appetite
- Nausea and vomiting
- Confusion

## The Five-Day Kidney Flush

**Throughout the day:** Drink a minimum of ten 8-ounce glasses (2 1/2 quarts) of distilled or purified water (distilled is best) throughout the day. The kidneys need water to cleanse efficiently, so drink, drink, drink your water!

**Upon Rising**

- Drink 1 cup herbal tea such as agrimony, marshmallow, juniper, or buchu. (These can be found at health food stores.) These diuretic herbs will help rid the body of excess water and benefit the urinary tract as well.
- Drink fresh juice such as Kidney Tonic (page 190) or Cranberry Water (page 190).

**Breakfast**

8:00 A.M. Choose one of the following (and a concentrated greens powder, as desired; see the Resources Guide):

1. Awesome Green Smoothie (page 191) or
2. One of the vegetable juice recipes (pages 298–303).

**Midmorning**

- Drink nettle tea (and kidney herbal supplement, as desired; see the Resources Guide).
- Drink the Cranberry Water (page 190).

**Lunch**

12:00 Noon

- **Days 1 and 5:** You may have a vegetable salad, raw vegetable sticks, or lightly steamed vegetables like broccoli or cooked artichoke. Or choose from any of the juice, smoothie, or raw soup recipes. For salad dressing choose from olive oil, lemon juice, avocado, garlic, and any spices or herbs. (You can combine all these ingredients or those you desire.)

- **Days 2 through 4:** Choose any juice, smoothie, or raw soup recipes from the recipe section. You will not be consuming any solid food on these days.

## Midafternoon

- . Drink the Cranberry Water (page 190) (and take a kidney herbal supplement, as desired).

## Dinner

6:00 P.M.

- **Days 1 and 5:** You may have a vegetable salad, raw vegetable sticks, lightly steamed vegetables like broccoli or cooked artichoke, raw-food dishes, and dehydrated veggies and dehydrated crackers. Or choose from any of the juice, smoothie, or raw soup recipes. For salad dressing choose from olive oil, lemon juice, avocado, garlic, or any spices or herbs. (You can combine all these ingredients or those you desire.)
- **Days 2 through 4:** Choose any juice, smoothie, or raw soup recipes from the recipe section, or have 1 cup Potassium-Rich Vegetable Broth (page 182). You will not be consuming any solid food on these days. Break the liquid diet on day 4 with a raw soup and dehydrated cracker, as desired.

## Evening

- Drink herbal tea (and take an herbal supplement, as desired).

# KIDNEY-CLEANSING RECIPES AND PRODUCTS

## CRANBERRY WATER

Mix 1 to 2 teaspoons unsweetened cranberry concentrate in 8 to 10 ounces water. (Unsweetened cranberry juice or concentrate can be purchased at health food stores.) Add a couple of drops of liquid stevia, if desired. (Do not use any artificial sweeteners, including Splenda.)

## NETTLE TEA

The herb nettles is used traditionally for kidney cleansing and support; it helps eliminate uric acid. Drink 1 cup of this tea each day.

## KIDNEY TONIC

1 cucumber, washed, or peeled
  if not organic
1 handful parsley
1 celery rib

1/4 lemon, peeled, or a handful
  of mint
1/2-inch piece gingerroot

Cut the cucumber in half and juice. Bunch up the parsley and juice it. Then juice the celery, lemon, and ginger.

**Note:** Cucumber, watermelon, cantaloupe with seeds, asparagus, lemon, kiwifruit, and parsley are all considered natural diuretics.

## AWESOME GREEN SMOOTHIE

*1 small to medium cucumber, washed, or peeled if not organic*
*2 cups spinach, washed*
*1 small to medium avocado, peeled, pit removed*

*1 tablespoon virgin coconut oil (optional)*
*Juice from 1 lime or lemon*
*Pinch or drops of stevia to sweeten (optional)*

Cut the cucumber into chunks, add to the blender, and blend well. Add the spinach and blend. Cut the avocado into chunks and add to the blender along with the coconut oil, if using, lime juice, and stevia, if using. Blend until smooth, and then pour into glasses or bowls.

SERVES 2 (Store the second serving in a jar for use later in the day.)

## KIDNEY-CLEANSING HERBAL SUPPLEMENTS

You may also wish to take an herbal supplement that will detoxify the kidneys. It is not recommended that you formulate your own combinations of these herbs, since they are not combined in equal amounts (see the Resources Guide). Look for the following herbs, which are cleansing to the kidneys, bladder, and entire urinary system:

- Agrimony
- Buchu
- Burdock root
- Gingerroot
- Gravelroot
- Hydrangea root

- Juniper berries
- Lobelia leaf
- Marshmallow root
- Nettles
- Parsley leaf
- Uva-ursi

### Kidney Detoxification Program: Summary

- Increase consumption of water, vegetable juice, and herbal tea to flush toxins.
- Follow kidney detoxification menu plan.
- Take herbal formulas and detox teas (use according to product directions).

# CHAPTER SEVEN

## *More Detox Programs*

Now that you have successfully completed your colon-, liver-, gallbladder-, and kidney-cleansing programs, you can move on to some special cleanses that will help address specific problems. The lung cleanse, skin cleanse, and lymphatic cleanse can be carried out at any time as a means of augmenting and facilitating the removal of toxins. The *Candida albicans*, parasite, and heavy-metal detox programs have specific protocols that must be followed carefully for optimum results.

For all the programs, follow steps 1 through 5 throughout the process.

- **Step 1:** Eat only whole, alkalizing, organic, non-GMO foods, and make 50 to 75 percent of the foods raw.
- **Step 2:** Remove as many sources of toxicity as possible.

- **Step 3:** Drink plenty of purified water (2 to 2 1/2 quarts per day).
- **Step 4:** Add fresh vegetable juices to your diet at least once or twice a day.
- **Step 5:** Complete periodic juice fasts for one to three days (except during a heavy-metal detox).

## The Lung Cleanse

The lungs are one of the five major organs of elimination. The lungs breathe in air, which principally contains oxygen, nitrogen, hydrogen, and carbon, then process it by extracting what the body needs to produce fuel from the foods we eat. The lungs then expel carbon dioxide gas, along with some of the toxic wastes that have been produced in the body. It is crucial throughout the cleansing process to keep the lungs functioning at peak efficiency. Use the following breathing exercises to assist your lungs in their capacity as organs of elimination.

### BENEFITS OF LUNG DETOXIFICATION

- Increases overall health of the respiratory system
- Improves oxygen assimilation
- Eliminates mucus

### DEEP CLEANSING BREATHS

Breathe deeply from your diaphragm by filling up your belly and upper chest (let your belly stick out as you breathe in); hold for a count of two, and then expel the air. This exercise can be done throughout the day; do a minimum of six times. Try to be conscious of your breathing, especially if you are anxious or under pressure, so you don't hold your breath.

## AEROBIC EXERCISE PROMOTES DEEP BREATHING

"Aerobic" means in the presence of oxygen. Add a program of aerobic exercise to your daily routine for lifelong health and wellness—the lungs and the entire body will benefit. Great aerobic exercises that promote deep breathing include brisk walking, snowshoeing, jogging, bicycling, hiking, aerobic dance, step aerobics, swimming, and rebounding. Find something you enjoy and have the energy to perform, and try to exercise outside as often as possible, as outdoor air is usually less polluted than indoor air. A walk or jog in the fresh air is also nourishing to your spirit.

## RELEASE EMOTIONS LIKE SADNESS AND GRIEF

Negative emotions, particularly sadness and grief, are known to inhibit or impede lung health. Holding on to grief, sadness, and sorrow often leads to shallow breathing and lung contraction. These repressed emotions become toxic, as they interfere with the delivery of nutrients and the removal of waste products through the lungs. (See chapter eight for more information on emotional cleansing.)

## THE THREE-DAY LUNG CLEANSE

1. Remove all dairy products two days before you begin your cleanse. Dairy products are quite mucus

forming. Your body must rid itself of mucus, so you
don't want to add in mucus-forming foods before
you begin cleansing your lungs.

2. Cleanse the colon the night before you begin.
Continue cleansing the colon during the three-day
lung cleanse.

For three days, follow this menu plan:

**Upon Rising**

Juice of 1 lemon mixed with 8 to 10 ounces of hot water and
a pinch of cayenne pepper before you eat breakfast. This will
help your liver to start working.

**Breakfast**

Ten ounces freshly made grapefruit juice.

**Midmorning**

Eight to 10 ounces carrot, cucumber, and celery (combined)
juice between breakfast and lunch. This juice combination
will help alkalize your body during your three-day detox.

**Lunch**

Twelve ounces potassium-rich green juice. Potassium is a
cleansing tonic. Combine carrots, celery, spinach, parsley,
and kale orchard. If you want something more substantial,
you can pour the juice into a blender and add an avocado to
make a green smoothie.

## Late Afternoon

One cup mucus-cleansing tea an hour before dinner. Combine rose hips, ginger, and peppermint. These herbs help alleviate stuffy noses, mucous buildup in the lungs, and congestion. This tea is readily available in most supermarkets and health food stores.

## Dinner

Ten to 12 ounces green juice such as the juice you had for lunch or a green smoothie.

## Before Bed

Twelve ounces unsweetened cranberry water. Mix several ounces of unsweetened pure cranberry juice with water. Rich in antioxidants, cranberry juice helps fight bacteria in the lungs.

You may also wish to take a lung rejuvenation herbal tincture several times during the day (see the Resources Guide).

### Herbs Used in Lung Detox

- Fenugreek seed—helps prevent inflammation and helps heal conditions such as bronchitis and sore throats
- Hyssop—prevents spasmodic actions, preventing and curing coughs and bronchitis
- Thyme—helps reduce mucus, prevents the growth of excess mucus, and acts as an expectorant
- Horehound—promotes relaxation of the bronchus muscles, increasing the production of beneficial mucus; acts as an expectorant
- Coltsfoot—helps heal acute bronchitis, annoying coughs and whooping cough due to spasmodic actions; acts as an expectorant

*(Continued)*

- Nettles—soothing for allergies such as hay fever and asthma
- Sage—contains healing properties for colds, sore throats, and tonsillitis
- Long pepper fruit—stimulates the lungs
- Lobelia—relaxes the lungs, preventing unnecessary stress, and promotes better breathing
- Extract of turkey tail mushroom—supports the lungs and helps remove excess phlegm
- Gingerroot—stimulates the lungs
- Sweet violet flower and leaf—supports the lungs

Additional herbs that are helpful: yerba santa leaf, osha root, usnea lichen, lomatium root, echinacea, goldenseal, myrrh gum, shitake mushroom, propolis, and licorice root.

## The Skin Cleanse

The skin covers the entire surface area of the body, making it the largest organ of elimination. It has many important functions, including the regulation of body temperature and the elimination of toxins through sweating. It aids all the other channels of elimination during the detoxification process, so it is vitally important that the skin's pores do not get clogged. There are a number of ways to cleanse and support the skin so it can function optimally.

The junk food, bad oils, fried foods, fast food, drinks, and chemicals we eat often show up on our skin. Pimples, blackheads, rashes, age spots, oiliness, wrinkles, and dryness are usually a result of what we put in our mouths. When we consume processed, high-sugar, preservative-laden, or fried foods, for example, the body must work very hard to get rid of the toxins, so it doesn't have much time to create new, healthy, vibrant skin cells. The organs responsible for toxin elimination—the colon, kidneys, and liver—become overwhelmed, so the body attempts to remove toxins and excess waste through the pores, causing clogging such as blackheads, whiteheads, pimples, redness, rashes, and skin irritation.

## SIGNS YOU NEED TO DETOX YOUR SKIN

- Acne, pimples, frequent breakouts
- Skin problems such as rashes, eczema, and psoriasis
- Sallow skin
- Gray skin
- Dull, lifeless-looking skin
- Large pores

# 8 Detox Steps to Radiant Skin

## WATER

Water is key to flushing out toxins. It not only delivers nutrients to your cells and keeps your kidneys functioning well; it aids in eliminating wastes and toxins. Without enough water to help the body flush out the wastes, the body becomes like a pool of poisons. This leads to many poor health conditions, including skin problems such as acne, rashes, and irritations. If you want glowing, healthy skin, you have to drink at least eight to ten glasses of purified water every day. Yes, that's water—in addition to your juices. Not diet soda. Not energy drinks. Not coffee or tea. Not a beer or a glass of wine. Water—clear, taste-less water. Many people believe that by drinking soda or any other liquid, they keep themselves hydrated. That is not true. In fact, many of these liquids I just mentioned are dehydrat-ing, and if you drink them, you need extra water. Water is the most fundamental aspect of your skin detox program—and all detox programs. If you don't drink enough water on a daily basis, the other recommendations won't help you as much.

## DRINK ANTIOXIDANT-RICH JUICE

Start your day with an antioxidant-rich juice such as the Skin Cleanser Cocktail (recipe follows). Antioxidants help protect the skin from environmental damage and prevent premature aging.

### SKIN CLEANSER COCKTAIL

*1 cucumber, washed, or peeled*          *1 handful alfalfa sprouts*
*  if not organic*                        *1 small handful fresh mint*
*1/2 bunch fresh parsley*

Cut produce to fit your juice feed tube and juice all ingredients. Pour into a glass and drink as soon as possible.
SERVES 1

## BREATHE

Choose exercises that promote deep breathing for at least thirty minutes every day. Any kind of exercise that gets you to breathe deeply will do—walking, jogging, step aerobics, dancing, gardening, biking, other sports...whatever you enjoy! The most important point is to increase your circulation and get rid of toxins through your lungs and by sweating them out through the skin.

## SKIN DETOX TEA AND HERBS

Drink 2 cups per day of Yogi Skin Detox Tea, which can be found at most health food stores. Alternatively, you can make your own blend. This special skin tea consists of 1 1/2 parts dried nettles, 1 part dried calendula flowers, 1 part dried red clover flowers, 1/2 part dried symphytum leaf, and 1/2 part dried lavender buds. (This skin tea recipe is from Shatoiya de la Tour. She recommends it for problems from acne and rosacea to eczema and psoriasis. It is also recommended for burn victims. You should be able to find these dried flowers and leaves at herbal shops or some health food stores, or you can order directly from DryCreekHerbFarm.com.)

To make the tea, boil 1 quart of water. Remove from heat and add 4 to 5 teaspoons of the herbal tea mixture. Steep for about half an hour and then strain.

## SKIN-CLEANSE HERBS

I recommend the skin and blood rejuvenation tincture (see the Resources Guide). I've noticed impressive cleansing results when I've taken it. This tincture contains the following herbs.

- Oregon grape root
- Sarsaparilla (Jamaican) root

- Stinging nettle leaf
- Burdock root
- Yellow dock root
- Hawthorn berries
- Chlorella
- Butcher's-broom root
- Bull kelp thallus
- Bee pollen
- Southern prickly ash bark

## DRY-SKIN BRUSHING

The outer layer of the skin, known as the epidermis, can become clogged with dead skin cells, thus inhibiting the natural elimination of toxic waste through the pores.

It's important to keep your pores unclogged. Dry skin cells accumulate on the outer layers of your skin and need to be scrubbed off. Keep in mind that mineral oil–based creams and lotions and wearing tight-fitting clothes can also cause your pores to clog. When your pores are clogged, your skin will look lifeless, dull, and rough.

Brushing the skin with a natural bristle or vegetable fiber brush facilitates elimination of this waste from the skin. Brushing the skin when dry helps open the pores, increase circulation, stimulate the lymphatic system, and eliminate dead skin cells. Cleansing your skin regularly will reduce stress on the liver and kidneys because there will be less toxic load on them if the pores are kept open.

You can purchase a natural vegetable fiber brush at your health food store. Do not use a synthetic brush, as it scratches the skin. Brush the skin every day when dry, before bathing or showering. This type of brushing is best done in the morning, as it can be too stimulating and can interrupt sleep if done before bedtime.

- Start with the bottoms of your feet, and then continue brushing up the legs using a circular motion. Always stroke toward the heart, gently but firmly.
- Use circular, counterclockwise strokes on the abdomen.
- Always move from the outside toward the center, starting with the hands and moving up the arms.
- Brush lightly around the breasts; do not brush the nipples.
- Brush the entire body for best results.
- Place sea salt on the brush to cause the pores to open more.
- Wash your brush every few weeks and let it dry.

Don't scrub too hard, but use enough pressure to make your skin feel clean and glowing. Then jump into a warm shower or bath. Try to avoid having a very hot shower or bath because really hot water tends to dehydrate the skin, especially in cold weather. If you want to really stimulate your whole body, model the Europeans by alternating hot and cold water in the shower. This stimulates the immune system.

## SWEAT: CONVENTIONAL AND INFRARED SAUNAS

Sweating is the body's natural means for regulating body heat. A sauna induces perspiration for therapeutic purposes, which causes toxins to be released through sweat. Sweat is produced from lymphatic fluid, and heat causes toxins to be released from the cells into the lymph. This process lightens the toxic load on the liver and kidneys by providing an additional channel for elimination of wastes that are released during the cleansing process.

Conventional saunas heat the air to fairly high temperatures, usually between 180°F and 235°F. These high temperatures increase the heart rate and can put a strain on the hearts of sensitive individuals. If it's difficult for you to stay in a conventional sauna, one alternative is the infrared sauna. Infrared heat is a form of radiant heat. In this type of sauna, the heat acts on only 20 percent of the air itself, whereas 80 percent acts on objects like your body. Infrared heat can be used at lower temperatures (110°F to 130°F), which enables it to penetrate more deeply and induce sweating without draining your energy or putting an undo strain on your body. Infrared saunas allow your body to secrete up to three times more perspiration than conventional saunas.

Infrared saunas have been shown to facilitate the removal of environmental toxins such as PCBs, pesticide residues, and plastic toxins, as well as heavy metals that are difficult to remove by conventional cleansing programs.

The effects of a sauna can be invigorating and energizing as your body's toxic load is lightened.

Be sure to drink a lot of water before and after using a sauna. You might also want to take a packet of Emergen-C Lite to replace electrolytes and get some extra vitamin C.

## THERAPEUTIC BATHS

If you don't have access to a sauna, you can create a therapeutic bath at home to help your body sweat. The hot bath brings toxins to the surface of the skin and opens pores so the toxins can be eliminated.

- Fill a tub with water that is as hot as you can comfortably tolerate, preferably filtered water (water filters for tubs and showers or the whole house are now widely available).
- Plan to stay in the tub for ten to twenty minutes for maximum benefit.
- Add therapeutic ingredients. Here are suggestions for different baths:
  - Epsom salts help neutralize the acids in toxins; they contain magnesium, which helps muscles relax, and sulfur, which aids in detoxification; 1 cup is a good start.
  - Ginger is a favorite of mine. You can juice fresh gingerroot and pour 1/8 to 1/4 cup ginger juice into the water. Ginger helps the body sweat and draws out toxins.
  - Baking soda and sea salt make a good alkalinizing bath; add 1 cup baking soda and 1 cup sea salt to hot water.

- You can also add 5 drops lavender essential oil (gentle antiseptic), 5 drops chamomile essential oil (anti-inflammatory and antifungal), and 5 drops lemongrass essential oil (skin revitalizer). Avoid lemongrass essential oil if you have sensitive skin.

## EXERCISE

Aerobic exercise such as walking, jogging, swimming, bicycling, racket sports, snowshoeing, step aerobics, dancing, and rebounding increases your circulation and induces perspiration, thus promoting excretion of toxins more efficiently through the skin. You can combine aerobic exercises with strength training like weight lifting. Increase the time and intensity of your workout so you sweat as much as possible. Shower immediately after a workout to remove the toxins so they will not be reabsorbed.

## THE JUICE-CLEANSE THREE-DAY DIET

To begin the skin detox, eat plenty of fruits and vegetables and drink at least 2 quarts (eight 8-ounce glasses) of purified water each day. Remove vegetable oils, caffeine, refined carbohydrates, alcohol, and sugar from your diet to begin detoxing the skin and receiving a more healthy appearance. A few days before the cleanse, change your diet to include as many raw vegetables and as much low-sugar fruit as possible. This change will mean that when you restrict your diet to juice only, it will be less of an adjustment.

Drink 1 to 2 quarts of fresh vegetable juice per day. Eat no solid foods.

Avoid soft drinks, energy drinks, coffee, and black tea. You may have herbal tea.

Since you won't be consuming any fiber during your juice cleanse, it is important to take fiber to stimulate your colon and prevent the toxins from being reabsorbed back into the body. An evening laxative tea or herbal supplement is effective to get things moving. Psyllium husk and bentonite clay are very good for drawing out toxins from the body.

How you break a juice cleanse is as important as the cleanse itself. It is best to start with a raw salad, green smoothie, or raw-food dish for a day. The next day you can try some lightly steamed vegetables with brown rice. Don't go straight back to meat and other animal products or typical American foods.

## Lymphatic System Cleanse

The lymphatic system is one of the supporting channels of elimination responsible for getting rid of toxins. It comprises a network of ducts, called lymph vessels, and carries lymph, a clear, watery fluid that resembles plasma. The lymphatic system consists of the lymph nodes, lymph vessels, lymphocytes, tonsils, adenoids, cisternae chyli (channels that receive lymph fluid from the abdominal cavity), thymus, and spleen. It is a wide-ranging drainage system that returns water and proteins from various tissues back to the bloodstream.

Since the lymphatic system does not have an active pump, it's dependent primarily on exercise and breathing to move the lymph through its many vessels. Breathing acts like a pressure pump to move lymph, and exercise causes muscles to contract, pushing against and squeezing the lymphatic vessels, thereby pushing the lymph along in a type of "milking action."

The lymphatic vessels function as the garbage collection system. They pick up the by-products of cellular respiration that have been excreted into the intracellular fluid and carry them through the body for elimination. Therefore, keeping the lymph moving freely through the vessels is a vitally important step in the detoxification process.

Many people have a congested lymphatic system and don't know it. Swollen glands are symptomatic of congested lymph nodes. In America, the lymphatic system is the most overlooked system of the human body. In Europe, stimulation of the lymph flow is a commonly prescribed medical treatment. Most health care practitioners in the United States seldom consider the lymphatic system's critical role in preventing illness or its importance in healing.

## SYMPTOMS OF A TOXIC LYMPHATIC SYSTEM

- Allergies
- Chronic sinusitis
- Eczema and other skin conditions
- Loss of energy
- Fibrocystic disease
- Chronic fatigue
- Repetitive parasitic infections
- Edema
- Inflammation
- High blood pressure

- Frequent viral infections
- Puffy eyes
- Bacterial infections
- Low back pain
- Cancer
- Balance problems
- Arthritis
- Headaches
- Cellulite
- Excessive sweating
- Obesity

**Follow the dietary recommendations for the skin cleanse (pages 206–207).**

## SKIN CLEANSING FACILITATES LYMPHATIC CLEANSING

Dry brushing, saunas, therapeutic baths, exercise, and drinking plenty of water all contribute to cleansing the lymphatic system. Drink 2 cups of Yogi brand Skin Detox Tea. In addition, add the following cleansing steps.

## DEEP BREATHING

Deep breathing changes the pressure differential from the abdomen to the chest and is one of the two ways that lymph is moved through the vessels. Use your diaphragm to fill up the belly and upper chest with air, hold for a count of two, and expel the air. Do this several times a day. Remember to breathe deeply throughout the day, and be sure not to hold your breath when you're tense.

## LYMPHASIZER

The lymphasizer, also known as the healthy swinger, is an excellent aid to your lymphatic detoxification because it will actively move the lymph and blood through the body. Dr. Shizuo Inoue developed this machine after observing the rhythmic, side-to-side movement of healthy, well-toned fish. This type of machine creates a wavelike motion up and down the spine as it gently massages the body and oxygenates muscles, tissues, and cells. It moves lymph through the lymphatic vessels so it can efficiently deliver its load of toxins to the organs of elimination.

It's very beneficial for those with circulation problems or diabetes, or those using steroids. With this machine, you can have a low-impact workout that requires no active movement. You can lie on the floor with your feet in the machine's grooves and in ten to fifteen minutes get aerobic benefits for your lymphatic system equal to a half hour of exercise.

The lymphasizer provides a simple exercise without applying any stress on the spine or other body parts. Simply lie down and the machine will move your body from side to side. This simple side-to-side motion maintains a proper energy balance and oxygen supply to the body. Regular use of this relaxing massage movement stimulates your body and achieves relaxation and stress reduction. An immediately noticeable sense of well-being arises from the massaging swing action.

Though this machine is a great addition for everyone, it can be excellent for the disabled, for anyone with hip, knee, or ankle problems, and for those who for other medical reasons are unable to even bounce slowly on a rebounder. (There are a wide variety of lymphasizers on the market. Some are very high priced. Be sure to see the Resources Guide for information and recommendations.)

## LYMPHATIC MASSAGE

Lymphatic drainage massage can be quite helpful in promoting lymphatic system detoxification. The massage therapist works on the muscles of the body that push against the walls of the main lymphatic system vessels, thus aiding in the movement of the lymph, which carries toxins to the channels of elimination.

## *The Candida Detoxification Program*

*Candida albicans* are usually benign yeasts (or fungi) that naturally inhabit the folds and creases of the digestive tract and the vaginal tract in women. They normally live in a harmonious relationship with beneficial intestinal flora, also known as probiotics. In healthy people, *Candida albicans* do not present a problem because they are kept in check by the friendly bacteria that also inhabit the gut.

These good bacteria, however, can be easily destroyed by the use of antibiotics and other medications, allowing *Candida albicans* to flourish. Other factors connected with our twenty-first-century lifestyle, such as diets rich in sugar, refined carbohydrates, and alcohol; the use of birth control pills; and stress encourage yeasts to grow.

Thought to affect more than forty million Americans, systemic infection with *Candida albicans* is now being recognized as a complex medical syndrome known as "chronic candidiasis" or "yeast syndrome." The yeast organisms attach themselves to the intestinal wall, where they compete with cells and ultimately the entire body for nutrients, thus creating nutrient deficiencies. They also release toxic by-products (their waste) that contribute to symptoms of yeast overgrowth. This overgrowth of yeast is believed to cause widespread symptoms in virtually every system of the body, with the gastrointestinal, genitourinary, endocrine, nervous, and immune systems being the most susceptible.

## SYMPTOMS OF CANDIDIASIS

- Athlete's foot
- Canker sores
- Chemical sensitivities
- Depression
- Digestive problems
- Dry, cracking skin on feet, hands, or elbows
- Ear and sinus irritation
- Fatigue
- Feeling "sick all over"
- Immune system dysfunction
- Intense itching
- Intense cravings for sweets, bread, and/or alcohol
- Jock itch
- Respiratory problems
- Ringworm
- Skin problems, including rashes that won't go away
- Thrush in the mouth or the genital area

- Toenail fungus
- Vaginitis
- Weight gain

If you think you may have a yeast overgrowth, take the Candida Questionnaire on pages 218–23.

## PREDISPOSING FACTORS

Chronic candidiasis has many predisposing factors, such as altered bowel flora; decreased digestive secretions; over-consumption of sugar, alcohol, and high-carbohydrate foods such as bread, pasta, or pizza; drugs (particularly antibiotics); immune dysfunction; impaired liver function; nutrient deficiencies; and underlying disease states. To simply go after the yeasts and kill them off, using natural or synthetic antifungal agents, will not get to the root cause of why you developed candidiasis in the first place. It's a lot like cutting leaves off a weed. It's vitally important to address all the factors that predisposed you to yeast overgrowth and get to the root of the problem so it doesn't return in the future.

## CORRECTING THE PROBLEM

In addition to using antifungal agents, it's very important to address the predisposing factors. Here's what I recommend.

### Follow a Candida-Control Diet

During a candida detox program, incorporate a healthy low-carb diet, such as the one in *The Coconut Diet*, which contains more than seventy recipes. I recommend virgin coconut oil because it contains fatty acids that help kill yeasts. Sugars are a primary food for yeasts. The early phases of the diet eliminate grains, fruit, alcohol, sugars, and other carbs that quickly turn to sugar, such as refined flour and starches, which *Candida albicans* is known to feed on. All natural sugars should also be eliminated when cleansing the body of yeasts. Milk and dairy products need to be omitted because milk lactose promotes overgrowth of yeasts. Also, all mold- and yeast-containing foods such as alcohol, cheese, dried fruit, bread, and peanuts must be completely avoided. Food allergens should also be eliminated. Candidiasis sufferers may need to avoid these foods for a number of months, as *Candida albicans* infections are known to be opportunistic and very difficult to overcome if the condition is systemic (meaning that the yeast has spread to areas outside the digestive tract). It's best to stick with this diet until you are symptom-free and yeast-free, which can be determined by a stool test. See the box on page 229, "Foods to Avoid During a Parasite (or Candida) Cleanse."

### Include Plenty of Virgin Coconut Oil in Your Diet

Research shows that the medium-chain fatty acids in coconut oil kill *Candida albicans*. Caprylic acid is one of the fatty acids in coconut oil that have been used successfully to fight candida. William Crook, MD, the author of *The Yeast Connection* and developer of the Candida Questionnaire, reports that many physicians have used caprylic acid successfully for yeast overgrowth and that it works especially well for those patients who have adverse reactions to antifungal drugs. Coconut oil also contains two other medium-chain fatty acids, lauric and capric acid, that have been shown to kill *Candida albicans*. A study done at the University of Iceland showed that "capric acid, a 10-carbon saturated fatty acid, causes the fastest and most effective killing of all three strains of *C. albicans* tested, leaving the cytoplasm disorganized and shrunken because of a disrupted or disintegrated plasma membrane. Lauric acid, a 12-carbon saturated fatty acid, was the most active at lower concentrations and after a longer incubation time." This study makes the case that all the medium-chain fatty acids in coconut oil work together to help you get rid of *Candida albicans*. (To order large quantities of virgin coconut oil for a significant savings, see the Resources Guide.)

### Assist Digestive Secretions

A major step in treating candidiasis is improving digestion. Gastric hydrochloric acid, pancreatic enzymes, and bile all inhibit the overgrowth of yeasts and prevent its penetration into the surfaces of the small intestine. Decreased secretion of any of these components can lead to a proliferation of *Candida albicans*. In addition, modern society offers numerous factors that decrease hydrochloric acid, including stress, food excesses, overconsumption of fats and proteins, and chemical use, along with aging (over fifty). Harmful emotions such as fear, worry, and anxiety also decrease gastric secretions.

Other conditions associated with low stomach acid include malabsorption, pernicious anemia, rosacea, eczema, anemia, food allergies, thyroid dysfunction, vitiligo, atrophic gastritis, *Helicobacter pylori* infection of the stomach, and gastric cancer. You can take the gastric challenge test to measure the amount of stomach acid you have. Most holistic doctors have the materials to perform this test.

Supplementation with hydrochloric acid (betaine hydrochloride), pepsin, pancreatic enzymes, and nutrients that improve bile flow is helpful in treating chronic candidiasis. The proteases (pancreatic enzymes) break down proteins and are mostly responsible for keeping the small intestines free of parasites (yeasts, bacteria, protozoa, and worms). (A deficiency in pancreatic enzymes is also one of the reasons some people experience excessive hair breakage, slow growth or loss of hair, or poor fingernail growth.) Supplementation should include betaine hydrochloride, digestive enzymes, and a lipotropic formula to promote bile flow (the formula should include choline, methionine, and/or cysteine). (See the Resources Guide for recommendations.)

**Support the Immune System**
A compromised immune system leads to yeast overgrowth, and *Candida albicans* infection promotes damage to the immune system. It's a vicious circle. Tests can document immune dysfunction, but they are expensive. A practical (and free) evaluation is to look at your health history. A history of viral infections including colds and flu, sinus infec-

tions, outbreaks of cold sores or genital herpes, prostatitis in men, and vaginal infections in women are indicative of immune dysfunction.

Supplementation with antioxidants, which include vitamins C and E, beta-carotene, selenium, and glutathione (found in abundance in vegetables and especially their juices), along with virgin coconut oil (to control *Candida albicans*), can be very helpful in improving immune function.

### Detoxify the Liver

Drs. Michael Murray and Joseph Pizzorno, authors of *The Encyclopedia of Natural Medicine*, say that improving liver health and promoting detoxification may be critical factors in the successful treatment of candidiasis. They note that damage to the liver is often an underlying factor in chronic candidiasis as well as in chronic fatigue. Studies with mice have shown that even slight liver damage causes *Candida albicans* to run rampant.

Chapter six outlines the liver detox program. It's best to complete a liver/gallbladder detoxification before embarking on the candida detoxification program.

### Take Probiotics

Probiotics, which are strains of beneficial intestinal flora such as *Lactobacillus acidophilus* and *Lactobaillus bifidum*, promote a healthy intestinal environment. It's very important that as you kill off the yeast, you replace the good bacteria. Choose a good probiotic supplement as part of your wellness plan.

### Take an Antifungal Compound

In addition to coconut oil, you may benefit from taking a yeast-killing agent such as an herbal supplement that contains thyme, garlic, fennel, black walnut, pau d'arco, burdock, and barberry.

### Drink Plenty of Purified Water

It is very important to drink plenty of purified water to flush your system as you kill off yeasts—aim for 1 quart of water for every 50 pounds of weight. It will help reduce die-off symptoms (discomfort as the yeast in your system dies) and will promote weight loss and good hydration.

## THE HERXHEIMER REACTION AND CANDIDIASIS

Be aware that as yeasts die, your symptoms may worsen for a short time or you may experience some reactions, such as headaches or diarrhea. Such reactions are known as the die-off effect, which is the result of the rapid killing of microorganisms and absorption of large quantities of yeast toxins, cell particles, and antigens. Hang in there. Your health will improve if you stick with the program. You'll be delighted with how you feel when you finally rid yourself of this obnoxious parasite.

## CANDIDA QUESTIONNAIRE

If you suspect you might suffer from candidiasis, William Crook, MD, has developed a questionnaire that you can fill out to determine the likelihood. The score evaluation is at the end of the questionnaire.

## SECTION ONE: History

There are different point scores for each question. Note the points and add them up.

| QUESTIONS | POINTS |
|---|---|
| 1. Have you taken tetracycline or other antibiotics for acne for one month or longer? | 25 |
| 2. Have you at any time in your life taken other broad-spectrum antibiotics for respiratory, urinary, or other infections for two months or longer, or in short courses four or more times in a one-year period? | 20 |
| 3. Have you ever taken a broad-spectrum antibiotic (even a single course)? | 6 |
| 4. Have you at any time in your life been bothered by persistent prostatitis, vaginitis, or other problems affecting your reproductive organs? | 25 |
| 5. Have you been pregnant one time? | 3 |
| Two or more times? | 5 |
| 6. Have you taken birth control pills for six months to two years? | 8 |
| For more than two years? | 15 |
| 7. Have you taken prednisone or other cortisone-type drugs for two weeks or less? | 6 |
| For more than two weeks? | 15 |
| 8. Does exposure to perfumes, insecticides, fabric shop odors, and other chemicals provoke mild symptoms? | 5 |
| Moderate to severe symptoms? | 20 |

9. Are your symptoms worse on damp, muggy days or in
   moldy places?                                            20
10. Have you had athlete's foot, ringworm, jock itch, or other
    chronic infections of the skin or nails?
    Mild to moderate?                                       10
    Severe or persistent?                                   20
11. Do you crave sugar?                                     10
12. Do you crave breads?                                    10
13. Do you crave alcoholic beverages?                       10
14. Does tobacco smoke really bother you?                   10

**Total score for section one**                         _____

## SECTION TWO: Major Symptoms

For each of the symptoms below, enter the appropriate score
in the points column.

If a symptom is occasional or mild, score 3 points.

If a symptom is frequent and/or moderately severe, score
6 points.

If a symptom is severe and/or disabling, score 9 points.

| SYMPTOMS | POINTS |
|---|---|
| 1. Fatigue or lethargy | _____ |
| 2. Feeling of being drained | _____ |
| 3. Poor memory | _____ |
| 4. Feeling spacey or unreal | _____ |
| 5. Depression | _____ |
| 6. Numbness, burning, or tingling | _____ |

7. Muscle aches                                    _____

8. Muscle weakness or paralysis                    _____

9. Pain and/or swelling in joints                  _____

10. Abdominal pain                                 _____

11. Constipation                                   _____

12. Diarrhea                                       _____

13. Bloating                                       _____

14. Persistent vaginal itch                        _____

15. Persistent vaginal burning                     _____

16. Prostatitis                                    _____

17. Impotence                                      _____

18. Loss of sexual desire                          _____

19. Endometriosis                                  _____

20. Cramping and other menstrual
    irregularities                                 _____

21. Premenstrual tension                           _____

22. Spots in front of eyes                         _____

23. Erratic vision                                 _____

**Total score for section two**                    _____


## SECTION THREE: Other Symptoms

For each of the symptoms below, enter the appropriate score
in the points column.

If a symptom is occasional or mild, score 1 point.

If a symptom is frequent and/or moderately severe, score
2 points.

If a symptom is severe and/or disabling, score 3 points.

| SYMPTOMS | POINTS |
|---|---|
| 1. Drowsiness | _____ |
| 2. Irritability | _____ |
| 3. Lack of coordination | _____ |
| 4. Inability to concentrate | _____ |
| 5. Frequent mood swings | _____ |
| 6. Headache | _____ |
| 7. Dizziness/loss of balance | _____ |
| 8. Pressure above the ears, feeling of the head swelling and tingling | _____ |
| 9. Itching | _____ |
| 10. Other rashes | _____ |
| 11. Heartburn | _____ |
| 12. Indigestion | _____ |
| 13. Belching and intestinal gas | _____ |
| 14. Mucus in stools | _____ |
| 15. Hemorrhoids | _____ |
| 16. Dry mouth | _____ |
| 17. Rash or blisters in mouth | _____ |
| 18. Bad breath | _____ |
| 19. Joint swelling or arthritis | _____ |
| 20. Nasal congestion or discharge | _____ |
| 21. Postnasal drip | _____ |
| 22. Nasal itching | _____ |
| 23. Sore or dry throat | _____ |
| 24. Cough | _____ |
| 25. Pain or tightness in chest | _____ |
| 26. Wheezing or shortness of breath | _____ |

27. Urinary urgency or frequency     _____

28. Burning on urination     _____

29. Failing vision     _____

30. Burning or tearing of eyes     _____

31. Recurrent infections or fluid in ears     _____

32. Ear pain or deafness     _____

**Total score for section three**     _____

Total score for section one     _____

Total score for section two     _____

Total score for section three     _____

**Total score for all sections**     _____

| RESULTS | WOMEN | MEN |
| --- | --- | --- |
| Yeast-connected health problems are almost certainly present. | >180 | >140 |
| Yeast-connected health problems are probably present. | 120–180 | 90–140 |
| Yeast-connected health problems are possibly present. | 60–119 | 40–89 |
| Yeast-connected health problems are less likely to be present. | <60 | <40 |

## The Parasite Cleanse

Parasitic infestation is not limited to third-world countries but is actually growing at an alarming rate right here in North America. A number of health care professionals believe that parasites are the cause of or a contributing factor to a number of disease conditions, such as cancer, intestinal problems, and chronic fatigue.

A parasite is an organism that feeds off another. In our bodies, parasites often feed on the undigested, putrefied food that collects in the gastrointestinal tract, mucus in the lungs, and waste in the lymphatic system. They may be found in any area of the body that is sick or weak, often because of toxic overload. These intruders are able to proliferate when the immune system is compromised. Although some parasites, such as worms, are large enough to be visible in the stools, especially during a detoxification program when they are killed and being expelled, most are microscopic pathogens that can be detected only by a specialized stool test.

Common sources of parasites include improperly washed vegetables and fruit, contaminated water, and undercooked meats. Parasites are often transmitted from pets and can be transferred from other infected persons, sometimes from restaurant workers who don't wash their hands. The overuse of antibiotics interferes with normal intestinal flora and contributes to parasites' proliferation.

Because parasites are difficult to detect and often hide in the lining of the intestinal tract or in other organs and spaces of the body, their presence and the problems they cause may go undiagnosed or misdiagnosed. Parasites cause damage directly to the body, and their acidic waste excretions contribute to additional body toxicity. Microscopic pathogens like yeasts, protozoa, fungi, worms, and bacteria disrupt our digestive processes and contribute to compromised digestion, which negatively affects the immune system and leads to compromised nutrition.

Some parasites can fool the body, causing it to behave as if they are a normal part of the tissue or organ, so the immune system will not go after them. When they have established their presence, they can make "Swiss cheese" out of parts of our bodies by perforating tissues. Worms can burrow into the intestines, lungs, liver, brain—almost anywhere in the body. They can erode, damage, or block certain organs or spaces by clumping together. They can even appear as cancerous tumors in areas like the brain, heart, or lungs.

Parasites pass metabolic wastes that are toxic. Many people have trouble disposing of these toxins, which are reabsorbed into the system through the intestines. Parasites also suppress the immune system, which leads to further degeneration, fatigue, and illness.

Some conditions that promote parasitic infections are excess mucus, an imbalance in the intestinal flora, chronic constipation, and a toxic internal environment.

Parasites feed on the nutrients that are meant to nourish us. In other words, our cells may be starving because of the nutritional deficiencies that result from parasitic infestation. Often people with parasites will overeat because they are constantly hungry. Their bodies are trying to make up for the nutritional deficit created by the parasites.

Toxic metabolic waste overloads and overworks the organs of elimination and taxes the central nervous system, causing a host of symptoms, such as chronic fatigue, mood swings, depression, and anxiety. Parasites can also penetrate the skin, causing itching. When tissue becomes inflamed from the parasites, the body's white blood cells step up in defense. This activity can cause skin rashes and food allergies. Parasites can collect in the sinuses and nasal cavities, causing sinusitis, headaches, and pain above the eyes. Parasites can also produce sleep disturbances such as insomnia, teeth grinding, drooling, and nightmares. Since they rob the body of the best of the nutrients, you get the leftovers—fat, sugar, and chemicals like preservatives. It is believed that many overweight people have parasites and as a result they are constantly hungry. This leads to overeating. Parasites can also cause muscle and joint pain.

### Symptoms of Parasitic Infection

There's a huge variety of parasites and numerous diverse symptoms associated with them. Many of these symptoms are common for other conditions. See your doctor for a stool test to confirm the presence of parasites.

- Abdominal cramping, pain, or bloating
- Constipation
- Diarrhea
- Burning sensations when defecating
- Fluid loss
- Poor absorption of nutrients
- Irritable bowel syndrome
- Blood sugar fluctuations
- Food cravings
- Tiredness and weakness
- Allergies

- Anemia
- Fuzzy thinking
- Headaches
- Loose, foul-smelling stools
- Loss of appetite
- Coughing
- Fever
- Vomiting
- Gas and bloating
- Digestive problems
- Explosive bowel movements very soon after eating
- Mucus in the stools

- Leaky gut
- Nausea
- Hemorrhoids
- Bloody stools
- Fatigue and chronic fatigue syndrome
- Low energy
- Lethargy
- Excessive weakness
- Dry skin and hair
- Brittle hair
- Hair loss
- Itchy nose
- Itchy anus
- Itchy skin
- Hives
- Allergic reactions to food
- Crawling sensation under the skin or the nose
- Rashes
- Weeping eczema
- Cutaneous ulcers
- Papular lesions
- Swelling
- Sores
- Mood swings
- Nervousness
- Depression
- Forgetfulness
- Restlessness
- Anxiety
- Slow reflexes
- Insomnia
- Grinding teeth while asleep
- Bed wetting
- Drooling during sleep
- Awakening several times during the night
- Weight gain
- Obesity
- Loss of appetite or uncontrollable eating
- Inability to gain or lose weight

If you suspect parasitic infestation, see your medical doctor or naturopath for a stool test (or you can order a test online; see the Resources Guide). However, if the parasites are localized in areas outside the colon, such as the brain, nasal passages, or lungs, these tests are often inconclusive.

## MY PERSONAL EXPERIENCE WITH PARASITES

Awhile back, I completed the full internal cleanse, which took about a month. Step 2 was a liver/gallbladder cleanse with a parasite-cleanse addition. The instructions said that if I saw any signs of parasites, I should complete another round.

I did see a couple of unwanted guests, so I completed round two. Again I saw a couple of parasites. So I did a third parasite cleanse. Again I saw a few parasites. I thought I'd better complete a fourth round just to make sure they were all gone. That's when it all broke loose, as they say! Unbeknownst to me, I had a colony of parasites in my nasal cavities and three in my right eye. They began dying off in record numbers in my nasal passages. This continued for several weeks. When it was over, I could breathe more clearly than I could remember in a long while. I could also smell things I had not smelled before. What an experience! I had no idea that a person could have parasites in their sinuses or nasal cavities. Years before I had completed a parasite cleanse and got rid of a large number of parasites from my intestinal tract that looked somewhat like white rice.

I encourage you to look at the list of parasite infection symptoms. If you have a few of them, I encourage you to embark on a parasite cleanse. (See the Resources Guide for recommendations.)

The program that follows has been highly effective in helping many people rid themselves of these destructive pathogens.

## EAT A WHOLE FOODS DIET

The standard American diet of processed, high-carbohydrate foods, junk food, and nutrient-deficient fare contributes to parasitic infection by causing a buildup of wastes and toxins. Parasites love sugar and foods that quickly turn to sugar, such as pasta, pizza, bread, rolls, and crackers. The diet of most Americans is loaded with these foods. The detoxification programs in this book will help cleanse and detoxify your colon, liver, gallbladder, kidneys, lymph, skin, and blood, which is an important step for parasite cleansing. You may need to continue with the parasite cleanse for several weeks or months, as parasites can often be difficult to eliminate because they reproduce rapidly. Avoid the foods listed in the following box.

### Foods to Avoid During a Parasite (or Candida) Cleanse

- All forms of sugar, even natural sugars like those from fruit—parasites feed on sugar
- Breads, pasta, flour products—these quickly turn to sugar
- All products with yeast
- Milk and dairy products—these contain milk sugar
- Beer, wine, and all other alcoholic beverages—they turn to sugar and contain yeast
- Cheese—this contains yeast and mold
- Dried fruit—this contains sugar and mold
- Peanuts and peanut butter—these have a high mold content
- Mushrooms—these are a type of mold
- Coffee, tea, and tobacco—these can acquire molds or yeast in the drying process (exception: pau d'arco tea is helpful in killing off yeasts)

Your diet should include an abundance of beta-carotene-rich foods, which are converted to vitamin A as needed in the body. Vitamin A increases resistance to tissue penetration by parasitic larvae. Beta-carotene-rich foods include carrots, sweet potatoes, yams, squash, broccoli, parsley, kale, spinach, dandelion greens, and other dark leafy greens. These foods can be made into juices or can be eaten raw, slightly steamed, or baked.

Avoid foods that irritate the gastrointestinal tract or cause gas and bloating, which interfere with nutrient absorption. Diligently avoid overeating because it puts a strain on the entire digestive system, especially the colon and the liver. Many protein-rich foods, such as meat and fish, or even vegan foods, such as beans, lentils, split peas, nuts, and seeds, can cause irritation or flatulence. Limit gas-producing foods during the parasite cleanse. However, sprouted nuts, seeds, and beans are easily digested and provide some protein. You may need to supplement your diet with natural free-form amino-acid protein powder during the cleanse. (Avoid soy protein powder since soy has many health-damaging properties.) Gluten-containing grains such as wheat, rye, oats, and barley may cause irritation to the intestinal tract if you are gluten sensitive, and if that's true for you, should be avoided.

## GARLIC

Garlic is a helpful treatment for the removal of parasites, especially common worms like roundworm, pinworm, and hookworm. Take two raw garlic cloves per day, finely minced. If you place the garlic on a teaspoon and swallow it with water, without chewing it, you won't taste it. Garlic is also available in capsules or tablets. The recommendation is 500 milligrams two to three times a day. Other helpful antiparasitic foods include onions, scallions, leeks, radish, kelp, raw cabbage, ground almonds, blackberries, pumpkin, sauerkraut, and fig extract.

## HERBS

A variety of herbs are available to help kill and expel parasites and worms. Green or black walnut hull tincture is used for parasites in the blood as well as in other parts of the body. For roundworms, the following combination of herbs is effective: green or black walnut hulls, wormwood, ground cloves, gentian root, ginger, and mandrake root. Pink root, also known as Indian pink, was used by Native Americans to kill intestinal worms, especially roundworms. For removing flatworms such as tapes and flukes, the following combination of herbs is effective: male fern, pumpkin seeds, pinkroot, wood betony, chamomile, and senna. Other effective herbs include oil of oregano, quisqualis fruit, artemisia, licorice root, torreya grandis nut, astragalus root, elecampane root, butternut bark, wild yam root, oleuropein, pau d'arco bark, cat's-claw bark, barberry root, shiitake mycelia extract 6:1, shiitake mushroom extract 8:1, southern prickly ash bark, and cloves. Grapefruit seed extract and enzymes such as bromelain, papain, and protease have also been shown to be helpful—the enzymes break through the mucous barrier that covers and protects the parasitic cysts. Grapefruit seed extract (found at health food stores) has also been shown to eliminate protozoa and fungus on contact. (See the Resources Guide for parasite-cleanse product recommendations.)

## AVOID ALL SUGARS

Sweets of all kinds, as well as sugar and sugar substitutes, should be avoided. As mentioned earlier, parasites love sugar and flourish on all forms of it. During your parasite detoxification, it is imperative that you not eat any sweets. Drinking a glass of water with lemon and a drop or two of stevia (an herbal sweetener found at health food stores) can often satisfy the craving for sweets until you regain your will to resist.

## CLEANSE THE INTESTINAL TRACT

Parasites cling to and feed off the mucus-encrusted layer of waste buildup in the intestinal tract. Therefore, your parasite detox will not be completely effective until the colon is thoroughly cleansed of this mucous layer. Otherwise, the parasites become embedded in this matter and hide out. Follow the colon-cleanse program on pages 143–50 for at least two weeks before beginning the parasite cleanse. It's also helpful to complete the liver/gallbladder detox before undertaking a parasite cleanse so all your principal organs of elimination are functioning optimally.

## DIGESTIVE AND SYSTEMIC ENZYMES

Digestive enzymes are necessary for the proper digestion of food. Unless your diet is primarily raw food, your natural enzyme levels may be insufficient for optimum digestion, so a good enzyme supplement will aid digestion and relieve the body of some of its burden of enzyme production.

Digestive enzymes are taken with meals to help digest protein, carbs, and fat. Protease, lipase, amylase, bromelain, and papain are examples of supplemental digestive enzymes. Systemic enzymes are different from digestive enzymes in that they are taken between meals, usually about two hours after eating, to clean up undigested proteins and help maintain healthy blood and tissue functions. (See the Resources Guide for recommendations of systemic enzymes.)

## The Thirty-Day Heavy-Metal Detoxification Program

Living in the twenty-first century exposes every one of us to contamination from heavy metals. These intoxicants pour into our environment from thousands of sources that contaminate our air, water, food, buildings, and gardens. Lead is a common heavy metal that has been in our environment for decades. It's found in the solder that seals food cans, in crops grown in lead-contaminated soil, in atmospheric lead from glass manufacturers, and in industrial lead from printers, smelters, and various other sources, as well as from leaded dust that is used in ceramic glazes. Although gas and paint no longer contain lead, many of us who grew up in that era still have lead in our tissues from exposure during the 1950s, '60s, and '70s.

Mercury levels have become so high in many of our oceans and lakes that it has contaminated much of the world's fish and shellfish. The mercury becomes more concentrated as you move up the food chain, so larger fish like albacore tuna, swordfish, and shark are often highly contaminated. Fish meal is frequently fed to chickens (unless they're fed a vegan diet), so poultry is an additional source of mercury. Another common source is dental fillings, which are an amalgam of mercury and silver, as well as vaccinations, which can contain the compound thimerosal (mercury is used as a preservative). We are exposed to cadmium from phosphate fertilizers, the burning of fossil fuels, and the gases that are released from zinc, lead, and copper smelters. Tobacco smoke is also a source of cadmium. Other types of heavy metals that may accumulate in our bodies from environmental pollution include arsenic, tin, copper, and aluminum. Heavy metals tend to accumulate in the tissues of the brain, kidneys, liver, fat cells, and immune system. They are not easily eliminated by the normal channels of elimination but tend to stay in our bodies for decades, often severely disrupting normal metabolic function and sometimes causing irreversible damage. Their effects can range from subtle symptoms to serious diseases, and because metals build up in the body over long periods of time, the associated symptoms are often misdiagnosed.

Removal of heavy metals can be a slow, difficult process, and during a detoxification program there is usually a redistribution of heavy metals within the body. To rid yourself of them, carefully follow the guidelines in this section during your detoxification program.

## Symptoms of Heavy-Metal Toxicity

- Chronic pain in muscles and tendons or any soft tissues of the body
- Chronic fatigue
- Malaise—a general feeling of discontent, fatigue, illness, and lethargy
- Brain fog—state of forgetfulness and confusion
- Chronic infections such as *Candida albicans*
- Gastrointestinal disturbance such as diarrhea, constipation, bloating, gas, heartburn, or indigestion
- Food allergies and intolerances
- Dizziness
- Migraines or headaches
- Visual problems
- Mood swings, depression, and anxiety
- Nervous system malfunctions—burning extremities, numbness, tingling, paralysis, or an electrifying feeling throughout the body

Because heavy-metal toxicity can produce symptoms that sometimes are mistaken for other chronic conditions such as chronic fatigue syndrome, depression, or multiple sclerosis, it's wise to discuss heavy-metal toxicity with a qualified health care professional who specializes in environmental medicine.

## EAT AN ALKALINE DIET

Step 1 of the heavy-metal cleansing program outlines the principles of an alkaline diet. It's extremely important during a heavy-metal detox that you eat a diet that is 70 to 85 percent alkaline (see the box "Acid Versus Alkaline Foods" on page 21). Include a variety of the cruciferous vegetables, such as broccoli, kale, cabbage, cauliflower, and Brussels sprouts, as well as plenty of leafy dark-green vegetables to provide extra minerals and calcium. Heavy metals can displace vitamins and minerals, so continue with your daily juicing.

Unlike in most of the other detoxification programs, you'll want to consume adequate amounts of protein. Consume 2 to 4 grams of meat, poultry, or fish once or twice a day. Choose grass-fed beef, organic free-range poultry and eggs, or wild-caught fish. Alternatively, you can use vegan protein such as beans, lentils, split peas, whole grains (exclude wheat), nuts, and seeds, either raw or sprouted. You can also supplement your diet with protein powder.

A heavy-metal detox is not the time for a fast. You need plenty of amino acids during this time. One reason is for the production of the antioxidant glutathione, a tripeptide (three amino acids linked together) that is important in liver detoxification and greatly facilitates the removal of heavy metals. The other important reason for adequate protein consumption is that amino acids bind to heavy metals, and fasting can break down protective protein layers, exposing metals, causing damage in the absence of adequate protein.

## DRINK PLENTY OF CARROT JUICE

Carrot juice contains vitamins, minerals, and phytochemicals that are especially needed as antioxidants during heavy-metal detoxification. Drink two glasses of carrot juice each day, and add veggies such as celery, cucumber, parsley, sprouts, and jicama, as well as any greens such as kale, spinach, and beet leaves. Flavor with ginger or with herbs such as cilantro.

## CILANTRO, GARLIC, CHLORELLA, AND CHLOROPHYLL

Cilantro has demonstrated an ability to aid in the removal of heavy metals from the body. Add it to salads, soups, juices, and salsas. Sulfur-containing foods such as garlic and onions also help combat heavy-metal toxicity. Chlorophyll and chlorella are also known to aid in heavy-metal detoxification. Use concentrated greens products, liquid chlorophyll, or chlorella.

## WATER

Drink eight to ten 8-ounce glasses (2 to 2 1/2 quarts) of purified water each day; alkaline water is quite beneficial.

## SUPPLEMENT WITH FIBER SHAKES

Drink one to two fiber shakes each day. You can make your own (see pages 147–48 in chapter five on colon cleansing) or purchase a commercial blend. It's also advisable to take an herbal formula for colon regularity once or twice daily. (These must be purchased. See the Resources Guide for recommendations.) The fiber will help absorb the metals, preventing them from being reabsorbed back into the system.

## DO NOT TAKE ENZYMES DURING THIS CLEANSE

Enzymes can remove the protein that carries heavy metals out of the body, exposing the metals and causing damage.

## SUPPLEMENTS

You should take a supplement designed to rid your body of heavy metals. One formula I've used contains andrographis, turmeric, hops, and zinc. Also, take a probiotic formula (a friendly-bacteria formula): two after each meal. (See the Resources Guide.)

## REMOVE MERCURY AMALGAM FILLINGS

Silver dental fillings are made from an amalgam of mercury and silver. The mercury can be released as a vapor during chewing or cleaning your teeth. The resultant release of mercury causes it to be deposited in tissues throughout the body. Mercury from dental fillings is one of the principal contributors to human exposure to inorganic mercury. Studies of people with mercury-containing dental fillings have shown an association between the number and size of the fillings and the amount of mercury found in their urine.

## IMMUNIZATIONS

Thimerosal is a preservative that is still used in a number of vaccines. It contains 49 percent ethyl mercury by weight and generally contributes to as much as 25 micrograms of ethyl mercury per dose. For decades mercury-containing vaccinations were given to infants on a regular basis. However, because of the danger to health, the Food and Drug Administration has recommended that thimerosal be removed from all pediatric vaccines. (It may still be in some; check with your physician.) Nevertheless, it is still routinely used in influenza vaccines. Before you get a vaccine or allow your children to be vaccinated, make sure the vaccine contains no thimerosal or any other mercury-containing compound. Thimerosal aside, there are numerous problems with vaccinations. Dozens of studies have confirmed the hotly contested findings of Dr. Wakefield, whose 1998 study suggested a link between the MMR vaccine, chronic bowel inflammation, and symptoms of regressive autism. The work of Dr. Natasha Campbell-McBride showed that chronic bowel inflammation resulting from abnormal gut flora can lead to symptoms of autism, as well as many other neurological and behavioral problems. A documented side effect of vaccination, including smallpox, rabies, pertussis, and MMR vaccine, is encephalitis (inflammation of the brain), which can lead to permanent brain damage and result in regressive behavior.

Such research was opposed to the many vaccine industry-sponsored studies that refuted this association.

In 2012 the Italian Health Ministry conceded that the MMR vaccine caused autism in a then nine-year-old boy. The Bocca family was awarded a fifteen-year annuity totaling 174,000 euros (just under $220,000), plus reimbursement for court costs. The judge ruled the boy had "been damaged by irreversible complications due to vaccination (prophylaxis trivalent MMR)."

## DETOX REACTIONS IN THE HEAVY-METAL CLEANSE

The thirty-day heavy-metal detoxification program can initiate cold or flu symptoms or other reactions such as headaches.

Cleansing reactions usually last only a day or two. The presence of detox symptoms simply means the process is working, so don't be alarmed or deterred. Soon the symptoms will pass as the toxins are eliminated and health is restored.

## THE SAUNA DETOXIFICATION PROGRAM

Sauna detox is a protocol designed to rid your body of harmful toxins that it cannot eliminate on its own. Some health professionals believe this is the only way to get rid of plastic toxins. Sweating this stuff out is the key. As your body heats up in the sauna, it increases circulation to even the smallest blood vessels and hard-to-reach areas. When you start to sweat, the body dumps toxins. They'll come from all over your body—blood, liver, kidneys, fat cells, joints, and tissues.

Numerous publications have shown that the sauna detox regimen has improved memory, cognitive functions, immune system strength, and general physical condition in different study populations.

## THE DIFFERENCE BETWEEN CONVENTIONAL AND INFRARED SAUNAS

Conventional saunas heat the air to fairly high temperatures, usually between 180°F and 235°F. These high temperatures increase the heart rate and can put a strain on the hearts of sensitive individuals. If it's difficult for you to stay in a conventional sauna, one alternative is the infrared sauna. Infrared heat is a form of radiant heat. This type of sauna heats only 20 percent of the air itself, whereas 80 percent directly heats objects like your body. Infrared heat can be used at lower temperatures (110°F to 130°F), which enables it to penetrate more deeply and induce sweating faster and without draining your energy or putting an undue strain on your body. Infrared saunas allow your body to secrete up to three times more perspiration than conventional saunas.

In one study performed by American researchers, the sweat of people using a conventional sauna was found to be 95 to 97 percent water, while the sweat of those using an infrared thermal system was 80 to 85 percent water, with the nonwater portion principally cholesterol, fat-soluble toxins, toxic heavy metals (such as mercury and aluminum), sulfuric acid, sodium, ammonia, and uric acid. This unusually high concentration of heavy metals and other fat-soluble toxins is not found in the sweat from normal exercise. Infrared saunas have been shown to facilitate the removal of environmental toxins such as PCBs, pesticide residues, and plastic toxins, as well as heavy metals that are difficult to remove by conventional cleansing programs. (See the Resources Guide for recommendations for a home infrared sauna.)

## THE SAUNA DETOX PROTOCOL

**Check with your physician.** Make sure your doctor gives you clearance for this program and contact your physician if any unusual effects occur.

**Start your day with a glass of fresh veggie juice or a green smoothie.** You may also eat protein such as a boiled egg.

**Take a multivitamin** that includes folic acid each day

of your detoxification program, just before exercising. Add 100 to 300 milligrams of potassium citrate and magnesium citrate for optimal results.

**Take niacin (vitamin B3) in increasing doses.** Niacin opens up even the smallest blood vessels and increases blood circulation throughout the body to aid in the cleansing process. Start with 100 milligrams before exercising, followed by an equal dose immediately after your sauna. Gradually increase the dose when it is clear how the niacin will affect your body. Do not use niacinamide or time-release niacin, and do not exceed the dosage limits recommended by your physician. The National Institutes of Health acknowledges niacin's role in breaking down fat and releasing toxins, but it also warns that niacin can be toxic at high levels. It is not appropriate for all individuals.

**Take digestive enzymes.** They will aid in detoxification as well as digestion.

**Exercise for fifteen to thirty minutes before using the sauna.** Exercise gets the blood circulating into hard-to-reach areas of the body where it can pick up toxins and eliminate them in the sweat. Choose an aerobic exercise such as fast walking, jumping on a mini trampoline, jogging, step aerobics, swimming, or biking to increase your metabolism, burn fat, and circulate your blood. This will aid in the detoxification process. Avoid a cooling-off period after your exercise. Go directly into the sauna while your body is still stimulated from the niacin, exercise, and nutrients.

**Spend three to four hours a day in and out of the sauna for a minimum of two weeks.** Start with fifteen minutes. Go naked in the sauna if possible. Then break for twenty to thirty minutes. Rest during your breaks. Return for fifteen minutes, and break again for twenty to thirty minutes. Take a warm (but not hot) alternating with cool shower and use a vegetable bristle brush to remove toxins and waste from your skin. Do not use soap. Repeat this process for two to three more hours. You will not be able to work full-time and complete this program.

**Eat lunch during a thirty-minute break.** Make sure your lunch is very healthy, for example, a big main-course salad. You may add some free-range or grass-fed animal protein to your salad.

**Drink purified water.** Be sure to drink a lot of water before and after a sauna. You might also want to take a packet of Emergen-C Lite to replace electrolytes and get some extra vitamin C.

**Take a juice break.** Have a vegetable juice during one of your thirty-minute rest breaks.

**Eat a very healthy, whole foods dinner** with lots of vegetables, especially the cruciferous veggies such as broccoli, cauliflower, Brussels sprouts, and kale. You don't want to put any toxins into your body when you're trying to eliminate them.

# CHAPTER EIGHT

## Mental and Emotional Cleansing

The last phase of your program is mental and emotional cleansing. A juice fast or colon cleanse will certainly detox and renew your body, but any physical cleanse will be greatly enhanced by also detoxing your mind and emotions. How many people do you know who are worried, fearful, anxious, pessimistic, irritated, or critical? Maybe some of these feelings apply to you. It's a stressful world that we live in, and it's difficult to avoid negative thinking. But there's a price to pay for these thoughts and emotions that don't serve us. We can learn how to replace them with positive, health-enhancing thoughts and emotions that contribute to our well-being.

Mental and emotional toxicity leads to chemical toxicity in the body and can have devastating physical effects. For example, unresolved issues, defeating toxic thoughts, and emotional baggage are often contributing factors to a variety of physical symptoms such as migraine headaches, fatigue, fibromyalgia, insomnia, multiple chemical sensitivities, poor immune response, and intestinal problems. Research also links toxic thoughts and emotions to serious illnesses such as cancer and heart disease, as well as to anxiety, panic attacks, and depression.

Cleansing these thoughts and emotions from our bodies and souls is as important to our health as detoxing pesticides and industrial chemicals from our tissues. "If we don't root them out, they can become imbedded in the soul," says best-selling author Dr. Christiane Northrup. "A thought held long enough and repeated often enough becomes a belief." And that belief causes a biological change in the body. For example, stress causes the adrenal glands to produce corticosteroids—hormones that weaken the immune system, glandular function, and other systems. Suppressed anger is one of the most toxic emotional responses of all and leads to chronic ill health and poor behavioral choices. Toxic thoughts and emotions are acidic and can create an internal environment for illness, pain, and diseases such as cancer.

When we can rid our lives of negativity, we can begin to create the health and lives we want. To cleanse toxic thoughts and emotions, we need both mental and physical action that can transform the effects of unhealthy neurochemicals that have built up in our bodies.

# The Hard Facts on Toxic Thinking and Its Effects on the Body

What we focus on mentally and emotionally becomes our experience. We may have entertained negative thoughts such as irritation, resentment, criticism, and judgment of others and ourselves for years and, consequently, they have become so habitual that we are unaware of them. They may even seem "normal," but negative thinking is not normal; it's physically destructive. Negative emotions like anger, hate, worry, fear, jealousy, irritation, and bitterness can make us sick and pave the way to life-threatening diseases. These emotions are transmitted to the entire body through neurons and neuropeptides that send messages for good or for ill.

Candace Pert, PhD, one of the foremost neurobiologists of our time and former chief of brain chemistry at the National Institute of Mental Health, has written extensively about the connection between emotions and neuropeptides. She and her husband discovered that neuropeptides, which are chemicals that affect mood and behavior, join the brain, glands, and immune system in a network of communication that can affect us on a cellular level.

Here's how it works: White blood cells have receptor sites for neuropeptides, and when our thoughts are negative, the messengers' (neuropeptides) communication can disrupt the health of our immune cells. Negative thoughts and emotions have been found to decrease T cell production and activity and to release stress hormones. Some neuropeptides can even trigger cancer cells to metastasize. Conversely, others help keep our bodies healthy.

Chemicals produced by toxic emotions lodge in our muscles, and we can experience neck and back pain or pain in other parts of our bodies. We can experience weakness or intestinal disturbances such as poor digestion, constipation, or diarrhea. The effects of negative emotions are also stored in the liver and kidneys and can disrupt their function and block proper pancreatic function. Unhealthy emotions can also cause cognitive inhibition, affecting our ability to comprehend, think, and make rational decisions. And traumatic memories may trigger allergic reactions. The list could go on and on, but the point to remember is that negative emotions are disruptive to the body, produce toxicity, and can be devastating to our health.

## The Mind-Body Connection

The mind-body connection, meaning the connection between thinking, emotions, and the health of the body, is not new. But we forget how powerful this connection is. There are distinct emotional and mental patterns associated with illness. The way you choose to use your mind, will, and emotions and the way you respond to your outer world have as much to do with disease as your diet, lifestyle, and environment do, and may even have a greater effect.

The body is a mirror of your thoughts, emotions, and beliefs. Every cell in your body has its own intelligence and is

able to listen to what you are thinking, feeling, and expressing. Your cells respond to each thought, every emotion, and
every word you say. Repetitive methods of negative thinking and suppressing negative emotions such as anger, resentment, and hatred, and even those that seem milder such as
irritation, annoyance, or frustration, can eventually manifest
as illness. Negative thinking is like a ticking time bomb waiting for the perfect conditions to explode.

Science has shown that when you are in a state of distress, your cells are not in harmony. When you operate in
stress and negative thinking, toxic chemicals are created, and
toxic chemicals promote sick cells. Once you are in this state,
you are prone to attracting viruses, harmful bacteria, parasites, fungus, and yeast such as *Candida albicans*.

More than any other factor, emotional stress weakens the
immune system, and you are less able to control everything
from parasites to cancer cells. Also, when you are stressed
or harboring unhealthy emotions, you tense up. This tension causes biological processes to be impaired. Nutrient
transport, cell respiration, detoxification, elimination, digestion, assimilation, hormone production, and brain function
become disrupted, leading to a gradual degeneration in the
body. But when you are in a state of balance—mentally, emotionally, spiritually, and physically—illness simply can't settle in your body.

Most people have not been taught how to deal with stress
or negative thinking and don't know how to live a balanced
life. Our society promotes drama, tension, stress, negativity,

and struggle, which makes natural, relaxed behavior nearly impossible. The secret to being free of the effects of all these unhealthy responses is to stop thinking, suppressing, and storing negative thoughts and emotions, find your divine purpose, learn to love all creatures, and live your life in a positive, joy-filled expression of who you really are.

## Transforming Toxic Thoughts

By detoxifying your physical body, you begin a process that will help you cleanse and transform your thoughts and emotions. As you pour fresh live juices and green smoothies into your body, they will push out toxic substances that have been stored in tissues, fluids, and cells. Emotions attached to toxic substances often surface when you cleanse, especially when you cleanse your liver. You can assist this process by allowing old thought patterns and emotions to come into full consciousness during detoxification and then release them and let them go. You may need to "dig up" others and release them so you can be free.

The first step in the process of letting go is to identify unhealthy thoughts. You may not be aware that some of your thinking, which may seem quite routine and normal, is actually toxic. You may have grown up in a negative family, and such thinking seems routine. Or maybe you've just thought critically or pessimistically for years because of circumstances in your life. This is not normal. Loving and positive thoughts are normal. Daily examination of your thinking is a process that can help you root out these thoughts and replace them with positive life-giving words.

Examples of negative thinking follow. Place a check by those that apply to you and add to the list as similar unproductive thoughts come to mind. After you have identified the negative thoughts, write a replacement thought next to each one. For example, if you checked *I hate my body*, write next to that something like *I have a unique body*. If you checked *I hate my nose*, you could write next to that *I have a very unusual nose. I could have been a memorable character actor.* Or next to *I have an incurable disease*, you could write *I have a health opportunity*. The most important thing is to listen to your heart and what it has to say.

_____ I hate my body.

_____ I'm too short / too fat / too skinny.

_____ I hate my nose.

_____ My hair is too curly / too straight / too fine.

_____ I'm ugly.

_____ I hate my thighs.

_____ I can't stand my life.

_____ My children don't love me.

_____ Nobody loves me.

_____ I'm never going to find a job I enjoy.

_____ I don't know if I'll ever find the right person to spend my life with.

_____ I'm never going to get well.

_____ I have an incurable disease.

_____ Nobody cares about me.

_____ I had a terrible childhood.

_____ I have a rotten marriage.

_____ I can't stand my job.

_____ There's never enough money to pay my bills.

_____ My life has no meaning or purpose.

_____ I'm lonely.

_____ I don't like where I live.

_____ I've never done anything exciting in my life.

_____ My mother / father treated me terribly.

_____ Nothing ever works out for me.

_____ I've always had a poor immune system.

_____ My life will never change.

This list could go on and on. The important thing is to do some self-assessment and recognize when your thoughts are either life enhancing or self-defeating. Your inner dialogue promotes health or disease. That's why it's so important to root out destructive thinking. For each negative thought you checked off on this list, you can practice letting it go. (See pages 255–62 for the letting-go exercises.)

Become aware of when you think negative thoughts. Here are some examples of how you can transform destructive, self-defeating thinking into positive thoughts. The next time a negative thought comes to mind, for example, "I hate my life," you can choose to think, "I'm working on finding (or fulfilling) my purpose, which is life-giving." If you think, "I'm never going to find a job I enjoy," you can say, "The right job awaits me; someone needs my skills and talents." If you think about your poor health and are tempted to think you'll never be healthy and full of life again, you can choose to think, "The juicing and cleansing I'm doing and all the good choices I'm making will produce better health. I'm getting better and healthier every day." Intercept all negativity as soon as it pops into your mind. You can say something like "I cancel or reject that thought" or whatever you choose to keep your mind from dwelling on this kind of thinking. As you practice this daily, you'll build a new habit of positive thinking.

## Transforming Toxic Emotions

The word "emotion" literally means "energy in motion." It's derived from a Latin verb meaning "to move." An emotion is a strong feeling such as love, fear, sorrow, or anger. Emotions move us; they generate complex mental and physiological reactions that produce change and affect our health on a cellular level. Emotional experiences get imprinted in brain cells, as well as in cells throughout the body, where they form patterns that influence our behavior and the chemistry of our bodies.

Emotional energy functions at a higher speed than thought. Scientists have confirmed that emotional reactions are recorded in brain activity before we even have time to think about them. We evaluate everything on an emotional level, and afterward, we think about it.

Being in touch with our emotions and learning to channel them in healthy ways, rather than stuff them or express them inappropriately, will lead to greater cellular and system health in our bodies.

Pure emotions such as anger and fear are not good or bad in themselves. We all need to feel fear so that we won't walk out in front of an oncoming car or wait too long to light a gas stove or fireplace. Sometimes we need to feel anger so that we can rise to the defense of someone or something in need, such as a child being abused, an animal being mistreated, or a country being torn apart. But we also need to let go of emotions that don't serve us, such as bitterness, resentment, blame, criticism, or irritation; they are never pure and always toxic.

Repressed traumas, which cause overwhelming emotions, can be stored for years in cells, tissues, and organs, thereby affecting their function. Trauma produces intense emotions that can become stuck in cells. Much has been written about sexual abuse and the traumatizing effects it continues to have on people who were molested as children. The same goes for physical abuse, verbal abuse, neglect, abandonment, isolation, rape, and many other traumas. What we know is that any form of trauma, whether emotional or physical, is stored in the body. When these traumas happen to a child, they are stored in the child's body and can cause the child to grow up with unhealed memories, pent-up emotions, and imbalanced neurotransmitters. And whether the trauma happened in childhood or adulthood, unless dealt with, cleansed, and let go of, the trauma can be like a ticking time bomb, just waiting for the right moment to explode. Holding on to traumatic events and unhealthy emotions creates problems because these events and emotions are stored on the cellular level. They need to be released for our well-being.

Releasing unhealthy emotional energy is essential for our cleansing process. Love, forgiveness, and letting go of demands that things in our lives be different are keys to neutralizing the effects of toxic emotions in our bodies. This can facilitate the cleansing process, promote physical health, and lead to joy and wholeness.

### Toxic Emotions: Contributors to Disease

- Anguish
- Anxiety
- Bitterness
- Blame
- Confusion
- Criticism
- Defilement
- Despair
- Discouragement
- Envy
- Fear (unhealthy)
- Grief
- Guilt
- Hate
- Humiliation
- Insecurity
- Irritation
- Rage
- Rejection of self
- Resentment
- Shame
- Sorrow
- Strife
- Unforgiveness
- Unhealthy or suppressed anger
- Worry
- Worthlessness
- Wrath

### Positive Emotions: Contributors to Vibrant Health

- Appreciation
- Contentment
- Curiosity
- Empathy
- Enthusiasm
- Gratitude
- Hope
- Interest
- Joy
- Kindness
- Laughter
- Love
- Optimism
- Peace

# Cleansing Negative Emotions: The Letting-Go Method

The Sedona Method, also called the release technique, is a simple yet powerful process that helps us release unwanted emotions that may be poisoning our bodies and souls.

The creator of this method, Lester Levenson, nearly died of a massive heart attack and was given just weeks to live by his physicians. During an intense period of self-examination, he came to believe that it was not the world or the people in it that were the cause of his problems. He acknowledged that his own emotional responses to events in his life had caused his health issues. Levenson discovered that he was capable of completely discharging all his negative emotions. As a result, his health and life flourished, and the Sedona Method was born.

This technique has undergone numerous scientific studies. Dr. Richard Davidson of the Laboratory of Cognitive Psychobiology at the State University of New York and Dr. David McClelland of the Department of Psychology and Social Relations at Harvard University conducted one such independent study. They concluded that the Sedona Method was highly effective in stress reduction. In a three-and-a-half-month follow-up study, dramatic reductions in stress were still present for participants.

Levenson found that people have three ways in which they deal with a feeling—they suppress it, they express it, or they escape.

When feelings are suppressed, we create an environment in which tension, anxiety, and depression can fester. This is very toxic to the body, and the most harmful way to deal with the emotions. Suppressed emotions create physical problems and behavior that is very unhealthy and sometimes uncontrollable.

Some people deal with emotions by expressing or venting them often. But even when an emotion is vented, it doesn't go away; it still needs to be dealt with. And after a blowup, for example, there's often an accompanying emotion of guilt. We are usually remorseful for our lack of control and, often, for the unkind words we spoke. All in all, expressing negative emotions is not a healthy way to deal with them either.

The third way people deal with their emotions is to escape, which may be by watching television, reading a book, surfing the Internet, eating, calling a friend, shopping, drinking alcohol, gambling, using recreational or prescription drugs, having sex, or smoking. But the emotions that are causing stress in the body are still there. Like the other two ways of dealing with emotions, escape does not work.

There is a healthy way to deal with our emotions. Many great teachers have taught this way throughout time. Release the feeling—simply let it go. (The technique follows.) Discharging the feeling is the healthiest way to deal with emotions. Laughter is one form of release. Most of us have had arguments in which, all of a sudden, we realize how silly the whole thing is and burst into laughter. At that point our bodies feel light and free. The emotion released was no longer in the body's tissues or contaminating our dialogue. Or we may cry and the falling tears help us release a heavy burden.

When we put the release technique into practice, it has a cumulative effect. We become more clearheaded, productive, and calm. Over time we can reach a state of imperturbability in which nothing can throw us off center. We can maintain our cool whatever the situation. We become more productive on the job, happier in our relationships, and at peace with our lives.

Here's how the technique is completed:

## STEP 1: FOCUS

Select a problem area in your life. Choose something with a lot of "emotional charge." Now allow yourself to become relaxed and calm.

## STEP 2: FEEL THE EMOTION

Ask yourself, "What am I feeling right now?" It really is important to tell the truth about your feelings. Listed below are six primary toxic emotions with many other emotions that are associated in those six categories. Identify the ones that apply to you.

**Anger:** Associated emotions that fall under anger are rage, aggression, annoyance, argumentativeness, bitterness, defiance, demandingness, disgust, irritation, frustration, fury, hate, impatience, jealousy, madness, meanness, outrage, resentment, spite, stubbornness, sullenness, vengefulness, viciousness, and violence.

**Apathy:** Associated emotions that fall under the category of apathy are boredom, carelessness, defeat, depression, discouragement, disillusionment, being drained, futility, hopelessness, being overwhelmed, powerlessness, resignation, and worthlessness.

**Fear:** Feelings subtyped under fear include anxiousness, apprehension, caution, cowardice, doubt, dread, foreboding, inhibition, insecurity, nervousness, panic, being scared, shakiness, being trapped, and worry.

**Grief:** Some subtypes of grief are feelings of abandonment, abuse, accusation, anguish, shame, betrayal, being cheated, embarrassment, helplessness, hurt, being ignored, being left out, being misunderstood, being neglected, rejection, and being sad.

**Lust:** This emotion yells "I want," and subtypes include anticipation, craving, demand, desire, deviousness, being driven, enviousness, frustration, greed, manipulation, obsession, ruthlessness, selfishness, and wickedness.

**Pride:** Some associated feelings under pride are aloofness, arrogance, boastfulness, cleverness, contempt, coolness, being critical, being judgmental, self-righteousness, rigidness, being self-satisfied, snobbishness, being spoiled, superiority, selfishness, being unforgiving, and vanity.

## STEP 3: IDENTIFY YOUR FEELING

Focus on what you are feeling at this time as you think about what has caused your hurt, fear, loss, rejection, or any other harmful response to an offense. Watch your body and identify what it's doing. Is your heart beating quickly? Are your eyes tearing? Do you feel nauseous? Is there tension in your muscles? Whatever is happening in your body is a clue to the emotions that need to be released.

Now select a word that best describes your feeling. When you have selected the word, find it in one of the six root-word categories. The process of release is most effective when the root emotion is released in its purest form along with all associated emotions. For example, it's more effective to release anger than it is to release annoyance. It's like pulling a weed out by its roots, rather than just cutting back the plant. When the root has been removed, the weed is gone for good.

## STEP 4: FEEL YOUR FEELING

Allow yourself to experience your emotions. Perhaps you feel angry. Allow yourself to be angry. Or perhaps you feel grief or sorrow. Allow yourself to be sad or to grieve. You may find yourself crying or sobbing. That is exactly what needs to happen at this time. It's okay to allow your feelings to permeate your body. This is not the time to stuff emotions or shut them down.

## STEP 5: COULD YOU LET GO?

While you are feeling the feeling, ask yourself the simple question "Could I let this feeling go?" One of the most freeing aspects of being an adult is being able to differentiate between our emotions and our true selves. That means that our emotions aren't us. They are simply energy moving through our bodies. Each of us has a "watcher or true self" that can observe the emotions as they flow through the body. It's this watcher that is asking the question "Could I let this feeling go?" We can view the emotion as a shadow image that has superimposed itself over who we really are. The feeling is not who we are, even though it may seem overwhelming.

Once we realize that we can feel the feeling and our true selves can ask a question at the very same time, we are able to see the possibility of letting the feeling go.

## STEP 6: WOULD YOU LET IT GO?

Once we realize that we can let the feeling go, it's possible for us to release it. We can ask ourselves, "Would I let it go?" This is where we need to be very honest. Sometimes we are simply too angry, hurt, or afraid to let it go at the present time. In that case we need to allow ourselves to continue feeling our feelings and not intellectualize or escape from them. There will come a time when we're ready to let the emotions go. We'll eventually get fed up with the effect they are having on our bodies, of the mind chatter, and of the disharmony they cause in our lives. When this happens we can truly say from the heart, "Yes, I can let this feeling go."

We may also answer no. Whatever you answer is okay; just repeat the process every so often until the answer is yes.

## STEP 7: WHEN WILL YOU LET IT GO?

Once we have acknowledged the possibility of letting this feeling go, the next question is "When?" Am I ready to let it go now, in ten minutes, tomorrow, next week? When will I let this feeling go? There will come a point when the answer is "Now! I'm willing to let this feeling go now. Right now! I don't want it anymore. I've processed this enough. I don't want to feel like this anymore. I want to be free."

## STEP 8: RELEASE

Once the decision has been made to let it go, the next step is simply to release it—let it go. You could picture it flying away like a dove or drifting off like balloons. Releasing your emotions will bring a wave of relief to your body. You may find yourself laughing, crying, or perceiving a sensation of chills going up and down your spine. Whatever the sensation, you'll feel lighter, as if a heavy burden has just been lifted from your body.

## STEP 9: REPEAT

Once you have released the feeling, it's time to observe your body. You may find that there are other emotions that need to be released. Simply go through the process as many times as needed. It's like peeling an onion. When one layer is gone, you may find that there's more to peel. Be patient with yourself and continue. It may take a period of time to completely cleanse your body and soul of all destructive emotions. Don't give up. This process works and creates a clean slate for you to begin the next phase in your cleansing and healing process.

Most people who use this technique find that their

energy skyrockets, their bodies are less tense, and they are more at peace with themselves and the world. The more the technique is used, the easier it becomes. People who practice this technique find that they are able to release emotions as they arise, making their family life or work environment much more congenial and peaceful.

## THE FINAL STEP

The more you practice the release technique, the more aware you may become of an underlying discontent and that you want more and more. There are two basic layers of want—wanting approval and wanting control. Until these underlying wants are released, there is always going to be an inner state of discontentment. The want for control or the want for approval will continue to underlie our emotions until they are released. When we release them, we'll have a wonderful sense of freedom!

## The Highest State of Being

The state of imperturbability is one of the highest states we can attain. This is a state where toxic emotions like irritation, resentment, bitterness, and worry are not allowed to remain in our consciousnesses. We can be in a place of serenity and peace all the time, a place where nothing can throw us off our courses or hinder our journeys toward wholeness. This is the state where our bodies can mend and heal from illness or disease, where we can conquer addictions and make life-giving choices consistently. It's important to remember that anytime we experience an emotion that is not loving, we go into a reactionary fight-or-flight survival response involving our reptilian brains, which inhibits our immune systems from working effectively. Letting go of negative thoughts and emotions opens up the heart, allowing it to beat in a coherent frequency, which allows us to respond in a proactive rather than a reactive way.

## *Forgiveness*

Forgiveness is healing for body and soul, whereas unforgiveness and an unforgiving spirit are detrimental to our health. Unforgiveness can lead to immune suppression and a host of diseases and can block the flow of energy in our bodies. Blocked or stagnant energy drains the body and taxes the immune system. When we hang on to unforgiveness, we hold ourselves in bondage. Though we may hold out on forgiving someone because we believe the wrongdoer must pay, and we'll not let him or her go in our minds and hearts until there is justice, it's our own bodies that pay the price, and we are wounded all over again. It's like drinking poison and expecting the person who gave it to you to die.

At times we may feel as if we're in control when we hold a grudge and unforgiveness in our hearts. We may be tempted to think that this can defend against the hurt, disappointment, or anger we feel about what was done to us, but the truth is that unforgiveness and attempting to control another person or situation actually make us powerless, and we are hurt in the end. A rattlesnake, if cornered, will sometimes become so angry it will bite itself. That is exactly what harboring unforgiveness and corresponding toxic emotions such as hate, resentment, or bitterness is like—a biting and poisoning of oneself. We may think that we're giving the person what they deserve by holding spite, but the deeper harm is to ourselves. Just how often should we forgive? As often as we experience unforgiveness. The biblical "seventy times seven" admonition concerning forgiveness is an Eastern idiom for infinite forgiveness.

Forgiveness and healing are linked. Forgiveness is the antidote to the emotional poison of the soul. Just as fiber carries waste out of the colon, forgiveness carries emotional toxicity out of the soul. Where hatred is a roadblock to health, forgiveness is the bridge to life and healing. For forgiveness to be complete and unconditional, we must be willing to let go of all stored emotions, such as bitterness, blame, grief, animosity, resentment, anger, irritation, or any other toxic emotion, and forgive from the heart.

### Forgiveness: A Key to Releasing Harmful Emotions

When we forgive others from the heart, not just the head, we free ourselves. In forgiveness, we're less driven to get even or to harm the one who hurt us. Forgiveness is positively linked to mental health and well-being. People who regularly forgive others report less depression, hostility, and anger. They are more hopeful and show higher self-esteem. Studies have shown that forgiving an offender leads to more positive emotions and a greater sense of control in one's life. In 2001, Charlotte van Oyen Witvliet and colleagues tested the physiological responses of undergraduates as they imagined real-life offenders in both forgiving and unforgiving ways. During forgiveness sessions, they empathized with the humanity of their offender and forgave the person. After the sessions, they reported less physiological stress, fewer negative emotions, more positive emotions, and a greater sense of control. The study found that empathy for the transgressor was a prevailing route to forgiveness.

To transform the emotions that have resulted from hurtful situations, and thus the memory of the hurt we've experienced, it can be helpful to go through some steps of forgiveness. You could address the following questions:

1. What do you know about the past of the person who hurt you? What was childhood like for the offender? Can you name a few things that could have contributed to this person's vulnerability? Remember that forgiving does not mean excusing someone's behavior. Also, make sure this person's hardships don't become your own.

2. At the time of the hurtful offense, what was life like for this person? Think about what he or she might have been thinking or feeling at this time. Was there a lot of pressure in this person's life? Was he or she feeling vulnerable?

3. What was your relationship with this person before the offense? How long had you known the person? Did you share any good times together? Name three positive things about this person.

4. As a result of the hurtful event, how might the offender be worse off now than before? What do you think life is like for him or her since the offense?

5. This person is a member of the human community. Though you do not need to welcome this person back into your life, can you see this person as part of the human family?

6. Has your view of this person changed in any way since answering these questions? Is there anything you can do to broaden your view of this person?

7. Can you let go of the offense and forgive this person?

CHAPTER NINE

# The A-to-Z Guide to the Nutrient Content of Foods

The following lists show the nutrient content of various foods. These lists can be used as a guide in planning your menu choices so you can meet your nutritional needs with food. As you read through the lists, note the various foods that you may not eat regularly but that are high in certain nutrients. One of the best ways to ensure that you are getting your daily requirements of vitamins and minerals is to eat a variety of different foods. Try to add something new to your menu every day. Most of the vegetables can be juiced (unless they are dense like avocados). Juicing further concentrates the nutrients and is a great way to obtain value from vegetables you might not normally consume, such as kale, Swiss chard, beet greens, or turnip greens. Combine these leafy green vegetables with carrots, beets, cucumbers, or celery and add some lemon, lime, green apple, or ginger for better-tasting juice.

While the values given in these lists can be useful in comparing the nutrient content of foods, absolute values for food nutrients will vary depending on such factors as the condition of the soil, type of fertilization, where the food was grown, how it was grown, the amount of processing or refining, and the method of preparation (cooked versus raw).

Keep in mind that studies show organic foods have a higher nutrient content and much less toxic contamination (especially from pesticides) than conventionally grown foods. Avoid genetically modified (GM or GMO) foods. Be especially mindful of soybeans and corn, and products made from them, as the majority of these crops are now GMO. Choose organically grown, as they are by definition non-GMO.

If you have questions about how to increase certain nutrients like vitamin C, potassium, calcium, or zinc, this guide provides valuable information to help you make wise choices. Some of the highest sources of these important nutrients are not widely known. For instance, almost everyone thinks that oranges and orange juice are among the best sources of vitamin C, yet vegetable sources like red peppers contain five times more vitamin C than oranges, and without the high fruit sugar. Another common example is the potassium content of bananas. For decades bananas have been advertised as one of the best sources of potassium, whereas vegetable sources like avocados, parsley, spinach, and Swiss chard are much richer in this mineral, and sunflower seeds and almonds contain almost twice the potassium bananas do. Instead of using whole milk for calcium, try some of the vegetable sources, such as kale, parsley, collard greens, and turnip greens—gram for gram, these contain about twice the calcium milk does.

When choosing seafood, keep in mind that many of our oceans are contaminated with various toxins, notably heavy metals such as mercury. Shellfish such as shrimp, crab, oysters, lobster, mussels, clams, and scallops are high in various nutrients, especially many of the minerals; however, these shellfish are also frequently contaminated with toxins, particularly because they are bottom-feeders that clean up garbage in the ocean. So be mindful of overconsumption of seafood. Additionally, be aware that mercury and other heavy metals tend to accumulate in larger fish because they are higher up on the food chain and heavy metals stay in their tissues. Eat sparingly of swordfish, albacore tuna, and shark. A safer alternative is to substitute smaller fish like trout, sardines, or salmon (wild-caught only). Use wisdom in all your food choices, balancing the nutrient values with awareness of the possible contamination from the many sources of toxicity in our environment.

## How to Use This Guide

The quantity of each food on the lists, which have been developed by the U.S. Department of Agriculture, has been standardized to 100 grams instead of common measurements.

This provides a more appropriate comparison between relative amounts of nutrients in foods and allows the foods to be ranked from highest to lowest. Remember that not all foods are consumed in 100-gram quantities as they may be very concentrated, for example, kelp, dulse, wheat germ, and brewer's yeast. These foods often appear at the top of the list, indicating them as concentrated nutrient sources. The following conversions may be useful to give you a better idea of what 100 grams of a food represents in common measurements.

| Approximate Equivalents | |
|---|---|
| 1 teaspoon fluid | = about 5 grams |
| 1 teaspoon dry | = about 4 grams |
| 1 cup milk or yogurt | = 245 grams |
| 1 cup leafy vegetable | = 90 grams |
| 1 cup root vegetable | = 135 grams |
| 1 cup nuts or seeds | = 140 grams |
| 1 cup sliced fruit | = 150 grams |
| 1 cup cereal grain, uncooked | = 200 grams |
| 1 tablespoon cooking oil | = 14 grams |
| 1 tablespoon honey or molasses | = 20 grams |

## The Order of This Guide

### VITAMINS

- Vitamin A
- Vitamin B complex
  - B1 thiamin
  - B2 riboflavin
  - B3 niacin
  - B5 pantothenic acid
- B6 pyridoxine
- B7 biotin
- B9 folic acid
- B10 para-aminobenzoic acid (PABA)
- B12 cyanocobalamin

- B15 pangamic acid
- B17 amygdalin
  (sometimes called laetrile)
- choline
- inositol

- Vitamin C ascorbic acid
  - Bioflavonoids
- Vitamin D
- Vitamin E
- Vitamin K

## MINERALS

- Calcium
- Chromium
- Copper
- Iodine
- Iron
- Magnesium
- Manganese
- Molybdenum

- Nickel
- Phosphorus
- Potassium
- Selenium
- Sodium
- Vanadium
- Zinc

## *Vitamins*

### Vitamin A

International units per 100 grams edible portion
(100 grams = 3 1/2 ounces)

| | |
|---|---|
| 21,600 Peppers, red chili | 6,100 Beet greens |
| 14,000 Dandelion greens | 5,800 Chives |
| 11,000 Carrots | 5,700 Butternut squash |
| 10,900 Apricots, dried | 4,900 Watercress |
| 9,300 Collard greens | 4,800 Mangoes |
| 8,900 Kale | 4,450 Peppers, sweet red |
| 8,800 Sweet potatoes | 4,300 Hubbard squash |
| 8,500 Parsley | 3,400 Cantaloupe |
| 8,100 Spinach | 3,300 Butter |
| 7,600 Turnip greens | 3,300 Endive |
| 7,000 Mustard greens | 2,700 Apricots |
| 6,500 Swiss chard | 2,500 Broccoli spears |

2,260 Whitefish
2,000 Green onions
1,900 Romaine lettuce
1,750 Papayas
1,650 Nectarines, prunes
1,600 Pumpkin
1,330 Peaches
1,200 Acorn squash
1,180 Eggs
1,080 Chicken
1,000 Cherries, sour red
970 Butterhead lettuce
900 Asparagus

900 Peppers, green chili
900 Tomatoes, ripe
690 Kidneys
640 Green peas
600 Elderberries
600 Green beans
590 Watermelon
580 Rutabagas
550 Brussels sprouts
520 Okra
510 Yellow cornmeal
460 Yellow squash

Vitamin A from animal sources occurs mostly as active, pre-formed vitamin A (retinol), while that from vegetable sources occurs as provitamin A (beta-carotene and other carotenoids), which must be converted to active vitamin A by the body to be utilized. The efficiency of conversion varies among individuals; however, beta-carotene is converted more efficiently than other carotenoids. Green and deep-yellow vegetables as well as deep-yellow fruits are highest in beta-carotene.

## Vitamin B Complex

### B1 *Thiamin*
Milligrams per 100 grams edible portion
(100 grams = 3 1/2 ounces)

15.61 Brewer's yeast
14.01 Torula yeast
2.01 Wheat germ
1.96 Sunflower seeds
1.28 Pine nuts

1.14 Peanuts, with skins
0.98 Peanuts, without skins
0.96 Brazil nuts
0.86 Pecans
0.74 Split peas

0.73 Millet
0.72 Wheat bran
0.67 Pistachio nuts
0.65 Navy beans
0.64 Beans, pinto and red
0.63 Heart, veal
0.60 Buckwheat
0.60 Oatmeal
0.55 Whole wheat flour
0.55 Whole wheat
0.48 Lima beans, dry
0.46 Hazelnuts
0.45 Heart, lamb
0.45 Wild rice
0.43 Cashews
0.43 Rye, whole-grain
0.40 Lobster

0.38 Cornmeal, whole-ground
0.38 Mung beans
0.37 Lentils
0.35 Green peas
0.34 Brown rice
0.34 Macadamia nuts
0.33 Walnuts
0.31 Garbanzos
0.25 Garlic cloves
0.24 Almonds
0.24 Lima beans, fresh
0.24 Pumpkin and squash
     seeds
0.23 Chestnuts, fresh
0.23 Soybean sprouts
0.22 Peppers, red chili
0.18 Sesame seeds, hulled

## B2 Riboflavin

Milligrams per 100 grams edible portion
(100 grams = 3 1/2 ounces)

5.06 Torula yeast
4.28 Brewer's yeast
0.92 Almonds
0.68 Wheat germ
0.63 Wild rice
0.46 Mushrooms
0.44 Egg yolks
0.38 Millet
0.36 Peppers, hot red
0.35 Wheat bran
0.33 Mackerel
0.31 Collard greens
0.31 Eggs

0.29 Split peas
0.26 Kale
0.26 Parsley
0.25 Cashews
0.25 Rice bran
0.25 Veal
0.24 Lamb, lean
0.23 Broccoli
0.23 Chicken, flesh and skin
0.23 Pine nuts
0.23 Salmon
0.23 Sunflower seeds
0.22 Beet and mustard greens

0.22 Lentils

0.22 Navy beans

0.22 Prunes

0.22 Rye, whole-grain

0.21 Beans, pinto and red

0.21 Mung beans

0.21 Black-eyed peas

0.21 Okra

0.13 Sesame seeds, hulled

## *B3 Niacin*

Milligrams per 100 grams edible portion
(100 grams = 3 1/2 ounces)

44.4 Torula yeast

37.9 Brewer's yeast

29.8 Rice bran

21.0 Wheat bran

17.2 Peanuts, with skins

15.8 Peanuts, without skins

11.3 Turkey, light meat

10.7 Chicken, light meat

8.4 Trout

8.3 Halibut

8.2 Mackerel

8.0 Chicken, flesh only

8.0 Turkey, flesh only

7.2 Salmon

6.4 Veal

6.2 Wild rice

5.7 Lamb, lean

5.6 Chicken, flesh and skin

5.4 Sesame seeds

5.4 Sunflower seeds

5.1 Beef, lean

4.7 Brown rice

4.5 Pine nuts

4.4 Buckwheat, whole-grain

4.4 Peppers, red chili

4.4 Whole wheat grain

4.3 Whole wheat flour

4.2 Mushrooms

4.2 Wheat germ

3.7 Barley

3.6 Herring

3.5 Almonds

3.2 Shrimp

3.0 Haddock

3.0 Split peas

## *B5 Pantothenic Acid*

Milligrams per 100 grams edible portion
(100 grams = 3 1/2 ounces)

12.0 Brewer's yeast

11.0 Torula yeast

2.8 Peanuts

2.2 Mushrooms

2.0 Soybean flour
2.0 Split peas
1.9 Perch
1.8 Blue cheese
1.7 Pecans
1.7 Soybeans
1.6 Eggs
1.5 Lobster
1.5 Oatmeal, dry
1.4 Buckwheat flour
1.4 Lentils
1.4 Sunflower seeds
1.3 Cashews
1.3 Rye flour, whole
1.3 Salmon, flesh
1.2 Camembert cheese

1.2 Garbanzos
1.2 Wheat germ, toasted
1.2 Broccoli
1.1 Brown rice
1.1 Avocados
1.1 Hazelnuts
1.1 Wheat flour, whole
1.1 Peppers, red chili
1.1 Sardines
1.1 Veal, lean
1.1 Turkey, dark meat
1.0 Black-eyed peas, dry
1.0 Cauliflower
1.0 Chicken, dark meat
1.0 Kale
1.0 Wild rice

## B6 Pyridoxine

Milligrams per 100 grams edible portion
(100 grams = 3 1/2 ounces)

3.00 Torula yeast
2.50 Brewer's yeast
1.25 Sunflower seeds
1.15 Wheat germ, toasted
0.90 Tuna, flesh
0.73 Walnuts
0.70 Salmon, flesh
0.69 Trout, flesh
0.66 Mackerel, flesh
0.60 Lentils, dry
0.58 Buckwheat flour
0.58 Lima beans, dry
0.56 Black-eyed peas, dry
0.56 Navy beans, dry

0.55 Brown rice
0.54 Garbanzos, dry
0.54 Hazelnuts
0.53 Pinto beans, dry
0.51 Bananas
0.44 Albacore, flesh
0.43 Beef, lean
0.43 Halibut, flesh
0.42 Avocados
0.34 Whole wheat flour
0.33 Chestnuts, fresh
0.30 Egg yolks
0.30 Kale
0.30 Rye flour

0.26 Turnip greens
0.26 Peppers, sweet
0.28 Spinach
0.25 Potatoes
0.24 Prunes
0.24 Raisins
0.24 Sardines
0.23 Brussels sprouts
0.23 Elderberries
0.23 Perch, flesh

0.22 Barley
0.22 Cheese, Camembert
0.22 Cod, flesh
0.22 Sweet potatoes
0.21 Cauliflower
0.20 Leeks
0.20 Molasses
0.20 Popcorn, popped
0.20 Red cabbage

## B7 Biotin

Micrograms per 100 grams edible portion
(100 grams = 3 1/2 ounces)

200 Brewer's yeast
60 Rice bran
58 Rice germ
57 Rice polishings
52 Egg yolks
39 Peanut butter
37 Walnuts
34 Peanuts, roasted
31 Barley
27 Pecans
24 Oatmeal
24 Sardines, canned

22 Whole eggs
21 Black-eyed peas
18 Almonds
18 Split peas
17 Cauliflower
16 Mushrooms
16 Whole wheat cereal
15 Salmon, canned
14 Bran
13 Lentils
12 Brown rice
10 Chicken

## B9 Folic Acid

Micrograms per 100 grams edible portion
(100 grams = 3 1/2 ounces)

2,022 Brewer's yeast
440 Black-eyed peas
430 Rice germ

305 Wheat germ
195 Bran
180 Kidney beans

145 Mung beans
130 Lima beans
125 Navy beans
125 Garbanzos
110 Asparagus
105 Lentils
77 Walnuts
75 Spinach, fresh
70 Kale
65 Filbert nuts
60 Beet greens and mustard
   greens
56 Peanut butter
56 Peanuts, roasted
53 Broccoli
50 Barley
50 Split peas

49 Brussels sprouts
45 Almonds
38 Whole wheat flour
33 Oatmeal
32 Cabbage
32 Figs, dried
30 Avocados
28 Coconut, fresh
28 Green beans
28 Corn
27 Pecans
25 Dates
25 Mushrooms
14 Blackberries
7 Ground beef
5 Orange

## B10 Para-aminobenzoic Acid (PABA)

As food sources with appreciable quantities of this nutrient
are few, a listing of the best sources of this nutrient is given
instead of showing relative nutrient amounts.

| | |
|---|---|
| Bran | Spinach |
| Cabbage | Sunflower seeds |
| Eggs | Wheat germ |
| Mushrooms | Whole milk |
| Oats | |

## B12 Cyanocobalamin

Micrograms per 100 grams edible portion
(100 grams = 3 1/2 ounces)

| | |
|---|---|
| 98.0 Clams | 17.0 Sardines |
| 18.0 Oysters | 6.0 Egg yolks |

5.0 Trout
4.0 Salmon, flesh
3.0 Tuna, flesh
2.1 Lamb
2.0 Eggs
2.0 Whey, dried
1.8 Beef, lean
1.8 Edam cheese
1.8 Swiss cheese
1.6 Brie cheese

1.6 Gruyère cheese
1.4 Blue cheese
1.3 Haddock, flesh
1.2 Flounder, flesh
1.2 Scallops
1.0 Cheddar cheese
1.0 Cottage cheese
1.0 Mozzarella cheese
1.0 Halibut
1.0 Perch, fillets

## B15 Pangamic Acid

As food sources with appreciable quantities of this nutrient
are few, a listing of the best sources of this nutrient is given
instead of showing relative nutrient amounts.

Apricot kernels
Corn grits
Oat grits
Pumpkin seeds
Rice bran

Sunflower seeds
Wheat bran
Wheat germ
Whole-grain cereals
Yeast

## B17 Amygdalin (sometimes called laetrile)

**High:** More than 500 milligrams per 100 grams edible
portion

Alfalfa leaves
Apple seeds
Apricot seeds
Bamboo sprouts
Bitter almonds
Cherry seeds
Elderberries
Fava beans

Macadamia nuts
Mung beans
Nectarine seeds
Peach seeds
Pear seeds
Plum seeds
Prune seeds
Wild blackberries

**Medium:** More than 100 milligrams per 100 grams edible portion

| | |
|---|---|
| Alfalfa sprouts | Lentils |
| Black-eyed peas | Lima beans |
| Boysenberries | Loganberries |
| Buckwheat | Millet |
| Currants | Mulberries |
| Flaxseed | Mung bean sprouts |
| Garbanzo beans | Quinces |
| Gooseberries | Raspberries |
| Huckleberries | Squash seeds |
| Kidney beans | |

**Low:** Less than 100 milligrams per 100 grams edible portion

| | |
|---|---|
| Beet tops | Green peas |
| Black beans | Lima beans |
| Cashews | Spinach |
| Commercial blackberries | Sweet potatoes, yams |
| Cranberries | Watercress |

### *Choline*

Micrograms per 100 grams edible portion
(100 grams = 3 1/2 ounces)

| | |
|---|---|
| 2,200 Lecithin | 245 Garbanzo beans |
| 1,490 Egg yolks | 240 Brewer's yeast |
| 504 Whole eggs | 223 Lentils |
| 406 Wheat germ | 201 Split peas |
| 340 Soybeans | 170 Rice bran |
| 300 Rice germ | 162 Peanuts, roasted |
| 257 Black-eyed peas | 156 Oatmeal |

145 Peanut butter
143 Bran
139 Barley
112 Brown rice
104 Veal
86 Molasses
75 Beef
75 Green peas
66 Sweet potatoes

48 Cheddar cheese
42 Green beans
29 Potatoes
23 Cabbage
22 Spinach
15 Milk
12 Orange juice
5 Butter

## Inositol

Milligrams per 100 grams edible portion
(100 grams = 3 1/2 ounces)

2,200 Lecithin
770 Wheat germ
500 Navy beans
460 Rice bran
390 Cooked barley
370 Rice germ
370 Whole wheat
270 Oatmeal
270 Brewer's yeast
240 Garbanzo beans
240 Black-eyed peas
210 Oranges
180 Peanuts, roasted
180 Peanut butter
170 Lima beans
162 Green peas
150 Grapefruit
150 Molasses
150 Split peas

130 Lentils
120 Cantaloupe
120 Raisins
119 Brown rice
117 Orange juice
110 Whole wheat flour
96 Peaches
95 Cabbage
95 Cauliflower
88 Onions
67 Whole wheat bread
66 Sweet potatoes
64 Watermelon
60 Strawberries
55 Lettuce
46 Tomatoes
33 Eggs
13 Milk
11 Beef, round

## Vitamin C Ascorbic Acid

Milligrams per 100 grams edible portion
(100 grams = 3 1/2 ounces)

| | |
|---|---|
| 1,300 Acerola | 38 Grapefruit and grapefruit |
| 369 Peppers, red chili | juice |
| 242 Guavas | 36 Elderberries |
| 204 Peppers, red sweet | 36 Turnips |
| 186 Kale leaves | 35 Mangoes |
| 172 Parsley | 33 Asparagus |
| 152 Collard greens | 33 Cantaloupe |
| 139 Turnip greens | 32 Green onions |
| 128 Peppers, green sweet | 32 Swiss chard |
| 113 Broccoli | 31 Okra |
| 102 Brussels sprouts | 31 Tangerines |
| 97 Mustard greens | 30 Oysters |
| 79 Watercress | 29 Black-eyed peas |
| 78 Cauliflower | 29 Lima beans, young |
| 66 Persimmons | 29 Soybeans |
| 61 Cabbage, red | 27 Green peas |
| 59 Strawberries | 26 Radishes |
| 56 Papayas | 25 Chinese cabbage |
| 51 Spinach | 25 Raspberries |
| 50 Oranges and orange | 25 Yellow summer squash |
| juice | 24 Loganberries |
| 41 Cabbage | 23 Honeydew melon |
| 46 Lemon juice | 23 Tomatoes |

### *Bioflavonoids*

As food sources with appreciable quantities of this nutrient
are few, a listing of the best sources of this nutrient is given
instead of showing relative nutrient amounts.

| | |
|---|---|
| Apricots | Blackberries |
| Black currants | Broccoli |

Cabbage
Cantaloupe
Cherries
Grapefruit
Grapes
Lemon juice
Oranges

Papayas
Parsley
Peppers
Plums
Prunes
Rose hips
Tomatoes

## Vitamin D

International units per 100 grams edible portion
(100 grams = 3 1/2 ounces)

| | |
|---|---|
| 500 Sardines, canned | 90 Sunflower seeds |
| 350 Salmon | 50 Eggs |
| 250 Tuna | 40 Milk, fortified |
| 150 Shrimp | 40 Mushrooms |
| 90 Butter | 30 Natural cheeses |

## Vitamin E

International units per 100 grams edible portion
(100 grams = 3 1/2 ounces)

| | |
|---|---|
| 216.0 Wheat germ oil | 11.0 Peanut butter |
| 90.0 Sunflower seeds | 3.6 Butter |
| 88.0 Sunflower seed oil | 3.2 Spinach |
| 72.0 Safflower oil | 3.0 Oatmeal |
| 48.0 Almonds | 3.0 Bran |
| 45.0 Sesame oil | 2.9 Asparagus |
| 34.0 Peanut oil | 2.5 Brown rice |
| 29.0 Corn oil | 2.5 Salmon |
| 22.0 Wheat germ | 2.3 Rye, whole |
| 16.0 Peanuts | 2.2 Rye bread, dark |
| 18.0 Olive oil | 1.9 Pecans |
| 13.0 Peanuts, roasted | 1.9 Rye and wheat crackers |

1.9 Wheat germ                0.88 Bananas
1.4 Whole wheat bread         0.83 Eggs
1.0 Carrots                   0.72 Tomatoes
0.99 Peas                     0.29 Lamb
0.92 Walnuts

## Vitamin K

Micrograms per 100 grams edible portion
(100 grams = 3 1/2 ounces)

650 Turnip greens             19 Green peas
200 Broccoli                  17 Whole wheat
129 Lettuce                   14 Green beans
125 Cabbage                   11 Eggs
89 Spinach                    8 Peaches
57 Watercress                 7 Beef
57 Asparagus                  6 Raisins
35 Cheese                     5 Tomatoes
30 Butter                     3 Milk
20 Oats                       3 Potatoes

## Minerals

### Calcium

Milligrams per 100 grams edible portion
(100 grams = 3 1/2 ounces)

1,093 Kelp                    296 Dulse
925 Swiss cheese              250 Collard greens
750 Cheddar cheese            246 Turnip greens
352 Carob flour               245 Barbados molasses

234 Almonds
213 Kale
210 Brewer's yeast
203 Parsley
200 Corn tortillas (lime added)
187 Dandelion greens
186 Brazil nuts
151 Watercress
129 Goat milk
128 Tofu
126 Figs, dried
121 Buttermilk
120 Sunflower seeds
120 Yogurt
119 Beet greens
119 Wheat bran
118 Whole milk
114 Buckwheat, raw
110 Sesame seeds, hulled
106 Ripe olives
103 Broccoli
99 English walnuts
94 Cottage cheese
93 Spinach
73 Pecans
72 Wheat germ
69 Peanuts
68 Miso
68 Romaine lettuce
67 Dried apricots
66 Rutabagas
62 Raisins
60 Black currants
59 Carrot juice

59 Dates
56 Green snap beans
51 Globe artichokes
51 Prunes, dried
51 Pumpkin and squash seeds
50 Cooked dry beans
49 Common cabbage
48 Soybean sprouts
46 Hard winter wheat
41 Oranges
39 Celery
38 Cashews
38 Rye grain
37 Carrots
34 Barley
32 Brown rice
32 Sweet potatoes
29 Garlic
28 Summer squash
27 Onions
26 Fresh green peas
26 Lemons
25 Cauliflower
25 Lentils, cooked
22 Asparagus
22 Sweet cherries
22 Winter squash
21 Strawberries
20 Millet
19 Mung bean sprouts
17 Pineapple
16 Beets
16 Grapes
14 Cantaloupe

14 Jerusalem artichokes
13 Tomatoes
12 Chicken
12 Eggplant
11 Orange juice

10 Avocados
10 Beef
8 Bananas
7 Apples
3 Sweet corn

## Chromium

Micrograms per 100 grams edible portion
(100 grams = 3 1/2 ounces)

112 Brewer's yeast*
57 Beef, round
42 Whole wheat bread*
38 Wheat bran
30 Rye bread
30 Fresh chilis
26 Oysters
24 Potatoes
23 Wheat germ
19 Green peppers
16 Eggs
15 Chicken
14 Apples
13 Butter
13 Parsnips
12 Cornmeal
12 Lamb chops

11 Scallops
11 Swiss cheese
10 Bananas
10 Spinach
9 Carrots
8 Navy beans, dry
7 Lettuce
7 Shrimp
5 Blueberries
5 Lobster tail
5 Oranges
4 Cabbage
4 Green beans
4 Mushrooms
3 Strawberries
1 Milk

**Note:** The values listed show total chromium content of these foods and do not indicate the amount that may biologically be active as the glucose tolerance factor (GTF). Those foods marked with an asterisk are high in GTF.

## Copper

Milligrams per 100 grams edible portion
(100 grams = 3 1/2 ounces)

| | |
|---|---|
| 3.7 Oysters | 0.3 Carrots |
| 2.3 Brazil nuts | 0.3 Clams |
| 2.1 Soy lecithin | 0.3 Coconut |
| 1.4 Almonds | 0.3 Garlic |
| 1.3 Hazelnuts | 0.3 Olive oil |
| 1.3 Walnuts | 0.3 Shrimp |
| 1.3 Pecans | 0.2 Chicken |
| 1.2 Split peas, dry | 0.2 Corn oil |
| 0.8 Buckwheat | 0.2 Eggs |
| 0.8 Peanuts | 0.2 Gingerroot |
| 0.7 Cod liver oil | 0.2 Millet |
| 0.7 Lamb chops | 0.2 Molasses |
| 0.5 Sunflower oil | 0.2 Whole wheat |
| 0.4 Barley | 0.2 Turnips |
| 0.4 Butter | 0.1 Apples |
| 0.4 Gelatin | 0.1 Green peas |
| 0.4 Rye grain | 0.1 Papayas |

Black pepper, thyme, paprika, bay leaves, and active dry yeast are also high in copper.

## Iodine

Micrograms per 100 grams edible portion
(100 grams = 3 1/2 ounces)

| | |
|---|---|
| 90 Clams | 37 Sardines, canned |
| 65 Shrimp | 16 Pineapple |
| 62 Haddock | 16 Tuna, canned |
| 50 Oysters | 14 Eggs |
| 50 Salmon | 11 Cheddar cheese |
| 46 Halibut | 11 Peanuts |

11 Whole wheat bread

10 Lettuce

9 Butter

9 Green peppers

9 Spinach

7 Milk

6 Beef

6 Cottage cheese

6 Cream

3 Lamb

3 Raisins

## Iron

Milligrams per 100 grams edible portion
(100 grams = 3 1/2 ounces)

100.0 Kelp

17.3 Brewer's yeast

16.1 Blackstrap molasses

14.9 Wheat bran

11.2 Pumpkin and squash
      seeds

9.4 Wheat germ

7.1 Sunflower seeds

6.8 Millet

6.2 Parsley

6.1 Clams

4.7 Almonds

3.9 Prunes, dried

3.8 Cashews

3.7 Lean beef

3.5 Raisins

3.4 Brazil nuts

3.4 Jerusalem artichokes

3.3 Beet greens

3.2 Swiss chard

3.1 Dandelion greens

3.1 English walnuts

3.0 Dates

2.7 Cooked dry beans

2.4 Sesame seeds, hulled

2.4 Pecans

2.3 Eggs

2.1 Lentils

2.1 Peanuts

1.9 Lamb

1.9 Tofu

1.8 Green peas

1.6 Brown rice

1.6 Ripe olives

1.5 Chicken

1.3 Artichokes

1.3 Mung bean sprouts

1.2 Salmon

1.1 Broccoli

1.1 Cauliflower

1.1 Currants

1.1 Whole wheat bread

1.0 Asparagus

1.0 Cheddar cheese

1.0 Strawberries

0.9 Blackberries

0.8 Red cabbage

0.8 Pumpkin

0.8 Mushrooms
0.7 Bananas
0.7 Beets
0.7 Carrots
0.7 Eggplant
0.7 Sweet potatoes
0.6 Avocados
0.6 Corn
0.6 Figs
0.6 Potatoes
0.5 Pineapple
0.5 Nectarines

0.5 Watermelon
0.5 Winter squash
0.5 Brown rice, cooked
0.5 Tomatoes
0.4 Oranges
0.4 Cherries
0.4 Summer squash
0.3 Papayas
0.3 Celery
0.3 Cottage cheese
0.3 Apples

## Magnesium

Milligrams per 100 grams edible portion
(100 grams = 3 1/2 ounces)

760 Kelp
490 Wheat bran, cooked
336 Wheat germ
270 Almonds
267 Cashews
258 Blackstrap molasses
231 Brewer's yeast
229 Buckwheat
225 Brazil nuts
220 Dulse
184 Filberts
175 Peanuts
162 Millet
160 Wheat grain, whole
142 Pecans
131 English walnuts
115 Rye
111 Tofu

106 Beet greens
90 Coconut meat, dry
88 Brown rice
88 Soybeans, cooked
88 Spinach
71 Eggs, dried
65 Swiss chard
62 Apricots, dried
58 Dates
57 Collard greens
51 Shrimp
48 Sweet corn
45 Avocados
45 Cheddar cheese
41 Parsley
40 Prunes, dried
38 Sunflower seeds
37 Barley

37 Common beans, cooked
36 Dandelion greens
36 Garlic
35 Raisins
35 Fresh green peas
34 Crab
34 Potatoes with skin
33 Bananas
31 Sweet potatoes
30 Blackberries
25 Beets
24 Broccoli
24 Cauliflower
23 Carrots
22 Celery
21 Beef
20 Asparagus

19 Chicken
18 Green peppers
17 Winter squash
16 Cantaloupe
16 Eggplant
14 Tomatoes
13 Cabbage
13 Grapes
13 Milk
13 Mushrooms
13 Pineapple
12 Onions
11 Oranges
11 Iceberg lettuce
9 Plums
8 Apples

## Manganese

Milligrams per 100 grams edible portion
(100 grams = 3 1/2 ounces)

3.5 Pecans
2.8 Brazil nuts
2.5 Almonds
1.8 Barley
1.3 Buckwheat
1.3 Rye
1.3 Split peas, dry
1.1 Whole wheat
0.8 Fresh spinach
0.8 Walnuts
0.6 Oats

0.5 Raisins
0.5 Rhubarb
0.5 Turnip greens
0.4 Beet greens
0.3 Brussels sprouts
0.3 Oatmeal
0.2 Cornmeal
0.2 Millet
0.19 Gorgonzola cheese
0.16 Carrots
0.15 Broccoli

0.14 Brown rice
0.14 Whole wheat bread
0.13 Corn
0.13 Swiss cheese
0.11 Cabbage
0.10 Peaches
0.10 Peanuts
0.09 Butter
0.06 Peas
0.06 Tangerines
0.05 Eggs
0.04 Beets
0.04 Coconut

0.03 Apples
0.03 Cantaloupe
0.03 Lamb chops
0.03 Oranges
0.03 Pears
0.03 Tomatoes
0.02 Apricots
0.02 Chicken breasts
0.02 Green beans
0.02 Whole milk
0.01 Cucumbers
0.01 Halibut
0.01 Scallops

Clover, ginger, thyme, bay leaves, and tea are also high in manganese.

## Molybdenum

Micrograms per 100 grams edible portion
(100 grams = 3 1/2 ounces)

155 Lentils
130 Split peas
120 Cauliflower
110 Green peas
109 Brewer's yeast
100 Spinach
100 Wheat germ
75 Brown rice
70 Garlic
60 Oats
53 Eggs
50 Rye bread

45 Corn
42 Barley
40 Fish
36 Whole wheat grain
32 Chicken
32 Whole wheat bread
31 Cottage cheese
30 Beef
30 Potatoes
25 Coconut
25 Onions
25 Peanuts

24 Lamb
21 Green beans
19 Crab
19 Molasses
16 Cantaloupe
14 Apricots
10 Butter

10 Raisins
7 Strawberries
5 Cabbage
5 Carrots
3 Whole milk
1 Goat milk

## Nickel

Micrograms per 100 grams edible portion
(100 grams = 3 1/2 ounces)

700 Soybeans, dry
500 Beans, dry
410 Soy flour
310 Lentils
250 Split peas
175 Green peas
153 Green beans
150 Oats
132 Walnuts
122 Hazelnuts
100 Buckwheat
90 Barley
90 Corn
90 Parsley
36 Whole wheat
35 Spinach
30 Fish
27 Cucumbers
25 Carrots
25 Rye bread

24 Eggs
22 Cabbage
20 Onions
20 Tomatoes
16 Apricots
16 Beef
16 Oranges
16 Potatoes
15 Cheese
15 Watermelon
14 Lettuce
13 Apples
12 Whole wheat bread
12 Beets
12 Pears
8 Grapes
6 Lamb
6 Pine nuts
6 Radishes
3 Milk

## Phosphorus

Milligrams per 100 grams edible portion
(100 grams = 3 1/2 ounces)

| | |
|---|---|
| 1,753 Brewer's yeast | 116 Fresh peas |
| 1,276 Wheat bran | 116 Mushrooms |
| 1,144 Pumpkin and squash seeds | 111 Sweet corn |
| | 101 Raisins |
| 1,118 Wheat germ | 93 Milk |
| 837 Sunflower seeds | 88 Globe artichokes |
| 693 Brazil nuts | 87 Yogurt |
| 592 Sesame seeds, hulled | 80 Brussels sprouts |
| 554 Soybeans, dried | 79 Prunes, dried |
| 504 Almonds | 78 Broccoli |
| 478 Cheddar cheese | 77 Figs, dried |
| 457 Pinto beans, dried | 69 Yams |
| 409 Peanuts | 64 Mung bean sprouts |
| 400 Wheat | 63 Dates |
| 380 English walnuts | 63 Parsley |
| 376 Rye grain | 62 Asparagus |
| 373 Cashews | 59 Bamboo shoots |
| 338 Scallops | 56 Cauliflower |
| 311 Millet | 53 Potatoes with skin |
| 290 Barley, pearled | 51 Okra |
| 289 Pecans | 51 Spinach |
| 267 Dulse | 44 Green beans |
| 240 Kelp | 44 Pumpkin |
| 239 Chicken | 42 Avocados |
| 221 Brown rice | 40 Beet greens |
| 205 Eggs | 39 Swiss chard |
| 202 Garlic | 38 Winter squash |
| 175 Crab | 36 Carrots |
| 152 Cottage cheese | 36 Onions |
| 150 Beef or lamb | 35 Red cabbage |
| 119 Lentils, cooked | 33 Beets |

31 Radishes
29 Summer squash
28 Celery
27 Cucumbers
27 Tomatoes
26 Bananas
26 Eggplant
26 Lettuce
26 Persimmons

24 Nectarines
22 Raspberries
20 Grapes
20 Oranges
17 Olives
16 Cantaloupe
10 Apples
8 Pineapple

## Potassium

Milligrams per 100 grams edible portion
(100 grams = 3 1/2 ounces)

8,060 Dulse
5,273 Kelp
920 Sunflower seeds
827 Wheat germ
773 Almonds
763 Raisins
727 Parsley
715 Brazil nuts
674 Peanuts
648 Dates
640 Figs, dried
604 Avocados
603 Pecans
600 Yams
550 Swiss chard
540 Soybeans, cooked
529 Garlic
470 Spinach
450 English walnuts
430 Millet
416 Beans, cooked

414 Mushrooms
407 Potatoes with skin
382 Broccoli
370 Bananas
370 Meats
369 Winter squash
366 Chicken
341 Carrots
341 Celery
322 Radishes
295 Cauliflower
282 Watercress
278 Asparagus
268 Red cabbage
264 Lettuce
251 Cantaloupe
249 Lentils, cooked
244 Tomatoes
243 Sweet potatoes
234 Papayas
214 Eggplant

213 Green peppers
208 Beets
202 Peaches
202 Summer squash
200 Oranges
199 Raspberries
191 Cherries
164 Strawberries
162 Grapefruit juice
158 Grapes

157 Onions
146 Pineapple
144 Milk, whole
141 Lemon juice
130 Pears
129 Eggs
110 Apples
100 Watermelon
70 Brown rice, cooked

## Selenium

Micrograms per 100 grams edible portion
(100 grams = 3 1/2 ounces)

146 Butter
141 Smoked herring
123 Smelt
111 Wheat germ
103 Brazil nuts
89 Apple cider vinegar
77 Scallops
66 Barley
66 Whole wheat bread
65 Lobster
63 Bran
59 Shrimp
57 Red Swiss chard
56 Oats
55 Clams
51 King crab
49 Oysters
48 Milk
43 Cod
39 Brown rice

34 Top round steak
30 Lamb
27 Turnips
26 Molasses
25 Garlic
19 Gelatin
19 Orange juice
18 Egg yolks
18 Lamb chops
12 Chicken
12 Mushrooms
10 Swiss cheese
5 Cottage cheese
4 Grape juice
4 Radishes
3 Pecans
2 Almonds
2 Cabbage
2 Carrots
2 Green beans

2 Hazelnuts
2 Kidney beans

2 Onions
1 Oranges

## Sodium

Milligrams per 100 grams edible portion
(100 grams = 3 1/2 ounces)

| | |
|---|---|
| 3,007 Kelp | 49 Turnips |
| 2,400 Green olives | 47 Carrots |
| 2,132 Salt, 1 teaspoon | 47 Yogurt |
| 1,428 Dill pickles | 45 Parsley |
| 1,319 Soy sauce, 1 tablespoon | 43 Artichokes |
| 828 Ripe olives | 34 Figs, dried |
| 747 Sauerkraut | 30 Lentils, dried |
| 700 Cheddar cheese | 30 Sunflower seeds |
| 265 Scallops | 27 Raisins |
| 229 Cottage cheese | 26 Red cabbage |
| 210 Lobster | 19 Garlic |
| 147 Swiss chard | 19 White beans |
| 130 Beet greens | 15 Broccoli |
| 130 Buttermilk | 15 Mushrooms |
| 126 Celery | 13 Cauliflower |
| 122 Eggs | 10 Onions |
| 110 Cod | 10 Sweet potatoes |
| 71 Spinach | 9 Brown rice |
| 70 Lamb | 9 Lettuce |
| 64 Chicken | 6 Cucumbers |
| 60 Beef | 5 Peanuts |
| 60 Beets | 4 Avocados |
| 60 Sesame seeds | 3 Tomatoes |
| 52 Watercress | 2 Eggplant |
| 50 Milk | |

The following foods contain large amounts of sodium chloride
added during processing and should generally be avoided:

Canned or frozen vegetables
Cured, smoked, or canned
   meats
Packaged spice mixes
Bouillon cubes
Canned fish
Commercial peanut butter
Ketchup, barbecue sauce
Potato chips, corn chips,
   pretzels, etc.

Luncheon meats
Salted nuts
Salted crackers
Canned or packaged
   soups
Processed cheeses
Commercial salad
   dressings
Meat tenderizers

## Vanadium

Micrograms per 100 grams edible portion
(100 grams = 3 1/2 ounces)

100 Buckwheat
80 Parsley
70 Soybeans
42 Eggs
35 Oats
30 Olive oil
15 Corn
15 Sunflower seeds
14 Green beans
11 Peanut oil
10 Carrots
10 Cabbage

10 Garlic
6 Tomatoes
5 Onions
5 Radishes
5 Whole wheat
4 Beets
4 Lobster
3 Apples
2 Lettuce
2 Millet
2 Plums

## Zinc

Milligrams per 100 grams edible portion
(100 grams = 3 1/2 ounces)

148.7 Fresh oysters
6.8 Gingerroot
5.6 Ground round steak

5.3 Lamb chops
4.5 Pecans
4.2 Brazil nuts

4.2 Split peas, dry

3.5 Nonfat dry milk

3.5 Egg yolks

3.2 Oats

3.2 Peanuts

3.2 Rye

3.2 Whole wheat

3.1 Almonds

3.1 Lima beans

3.1 Soy lecithin

3.0 Walnuts

2.9 Sardines

2.6 Chicken

2.5 Buckwheat

2.4 Hazelnuts

1.9 Clams

1.7 Anchovies

1.7 Haddock

1.7 Tuna

1.6 Green peas

1.5 Shrimp

1.2 Turnips

0.9 Parsley

0.9 Potatoes

0.6 Garlic

0.5 Carrots

0.5 Whole wheat bread

0.4 Black beans

0.4 Corn

0.4 Pork chops

0.4 Raw milk

0.3 Grape juice

0.3 Olive oil

0.3 Cauliflower

0.2 Butter

0.2 Cabbage

0.2 Lentils

0.2 Lettuce

0.2 Spinach

0.1 Cucumbers

0.1 String beans

0.1 Tangerines

0.1 Yams

Black pepper, paprika, mustard, chili powder, thyme, and cinnamon are also high in zinc.

CHAPTER TEN

# Recipes for Fasting and Detoxing

Most of the recipes here use vegetables, herbs, nuts, and seeds, plus nut or seed milk for the smoothies. A few recipes contain half of a low-sugar apple or pear for flavor. It's a healthful choice to avoid fruit juice as much as possible, since it contains too much fruit sugar and some can be acidic. The goal in the detox programs and maintenance diet is to alkalinize your body. When you do choose to add a little fruit for flavor, make sure it is low in sugar and always diluted with lots of vegetable juice.

| Low-Sugar Fruit | |
| --- | --- |
| Lemons | Green apples |
| Berries | Grapefruit |
| Limes | Pears |

# *Vegetable Juice Recipes*

Nearly all these recipes say to drink as soon as possible so
that you will get the maximum nutritional benefit. But if
you can't drink your juice right away or you need to make
it ahead of time, you can store it in a cold place such as the
refrigerator or in a thermos. Juice will last about 24 hours.
You will lose some nutrients this way, but it is still going to
give you a lot of nutrients. You can also freeze juice, and the
same information applies to frozen juice. Also, you can juice
all seeds that are soft; all hard pits must be removed.

## MORNING ENERGY

*3 to 4 carrots, scrubbed well,
    tops removed, ends trimmed
1 cucumber, washed, or peeled
    if not organic
1/2 beet, scrubbed well (may*

*include stem and 1 or 2
    leaves)
1/2 lemon, peeled
1-inch chunk gingerroot,
    scrubbed, or peeled if old*

Cut the produce to fit your juicer's feed tube. Juice all the ingredients and stir. Pour into a glass and drink as soon as possible.
SERVES 1 TO 2

## BEET-CUCUMBER CLEANSING COCKTAIL

*1 cucumber, washed, or peeled
    if not organic
3 carrots, scrubbed well, tops
    removed, ends trimmed
1 beet, scrubbed well, with stem
    and 1 or 2 leaves*

*2 celery ribs
1 handful parsley
1- to 2-inch chunk gingerroot,
    scrubbed, or peeled if old
1/2 lemon, peeled*

Cut the produce to fit your juicer's feed tube. Juice all the ingredients and stir. Pour into a glass and drink as soon as possible.

SERVES 1 TO 2

## SPRING CLEANSING COCKTAIL

Asparagus is a natural diuretic, which helps flush toxins from the body and promotes kidney cleansing.

> *1 vine-ripened tomato*     ·      *8 asparagus stalks*
> *1 cucumber, washed, or peeled*     *1/2 lemon, peeled*
>    *if not organic*

Cut the produce to fit your juicer's feed tube. Juice all the ingredients and stir. Pour into a glass and drink as soon as possible.

SERVES 1 TO 2

## LIVER-CLEANSING COCKTAIL

Dandelion juice is a traditional remedy for cleansing the liver.

> *1 handful dandelion greens*     *1/2 cucumber, washed, or*
> *3 to 4 carrots, scrubbed well,*     *peeled if not organic*
>    *tops removed, ends trimmed*     *1/2 lemon, peeled*

Bunch up the dandelion greens. Cut the produce to fit your juicer's feed tube. Tuck the greens in the feed tube and push through with one of the carrots. Juice the remaining ingredients, finishing with a carrot. Stir the juice, pour into a glass, and drink as soon as possible.

SERVES 1

## CUCUMBER REFRESHER

1 cucumber, washed, or peeled          1/2 lemon, peeled
   if not organic

Cut the produce to fit your juicer's feed tube. Juice all the ingredients and stir. Pour into a glass and drink as soon as possible.

SERVES 1

## DINO DELIGHT

1 cucumber, washed, or peeled          1/2 lemon, with peel, seeded
   if not organic                         (use only organic)
2 to 3 celery ribs, leaves             1-inch chunk gingerroot,
   included if desired                    scrubbed, or peeled if old
3 leaves Dinosaur kale

Cut the produce to fit your juicer's feed tube. Juice all the ingredients and stir. Pour into a glass and drink as soon as possible.

SERVES 1 TO 2

## THE ORIENT EXPRESS

2-by-4- or 5-inch chunk of             1 daikon radish, trimmed and
   jicama, scrubbed well or               scrubbed
   peeled                              1-inch chunk gingerroot,
2 to 3 carrots, scrubbed well,            scrubbed, or peeled if old
   tops removed, ends trimmed

Cut the produce to fit your juicer's feed tube. Juice all the ingredients and stir. Pour into a glass and drink as soon as possible.

SERVES 1

## SALSA IN A GLASS

1 medium vine-ripened tomato
1/2 cucumber, peeled
1 small handful cilantro

1/2 lime, peeled
Dash of hot sauce (optional)

Cut the produce to fit your juicer's feed tube. Juice all the ingredients and stir. Pour into a glass and drink as soon as possible.
SERVES 1

## SPICY TOMATO

2 medium vine-ripened
  tomatoes
2 dark green lettuce leaves

2 radishes, scrubbed
4 sprigs parsley
1/2 lime or lemon, peeled

Cut the produce to fit your juicer's feed tube. Juice all the ingredients and stir. Pour into a glass and drink as soon as possible.
SERVES 1

## TOMATO FLORENTINE

2 vine-ripened tomatoes
4 to 5 sprigs basil

1 large handful spinach
1/2 lemon, peeled

Juice one of the tomatoes. Wrap the basil in several spinach leaves. Turn off the juicer and add the spinach and basil. Turn the juicer back on and gently pulse to juice them. Juice the remaining tomato and lemon. Stir the juice, pour into a glass, and drink as soon as possible.
SERVES 1

## CABBAGE COCKTAIL

1/4 small head green cabbage
3 carrots, scrubbed well, tops
  removed, ends trimmed

4 celery ribs, with leaves if
  desired

Cut the produce to fit your juicer's feed tube. Juice all the ingredients and stir. Pour into a glass and drink as soon as possible.
SERVES 1

## SPINACH POWER

1/2 cucumber, washed, or
    peeled if not organic
3 carrots, scrubbed well, tops
    removed, ends trimmed
2 celery ribs, with leaves if
    desired

1/2 beet, scrubbed well (may
    include stem and 1 to 2
    leaves)
1 small handful parsley
1/2 lemon, peeled
1 large handful spinach

Cut the produce to fit your juicer's feed tube. Juice all the ingredients and stir. Pour into a glass and drink as soon as possible.
SERVES 1 TO 2

## SUPER GREEN DRINK

1 cucumber, washed, or peeled
    if not organic
1 large handful sunflower
    sprouts
1 small handful buckwheat
    sprouts

1 small handful clover
    sprouts
1 large handful spinach

Cut the cucumber to fit your juicer's feed tube. Juice part of the cucumber first. Bunch up the sprouts and wrap them in the spinach leaves. Turn off the juicer and add the sprouts and spinach. Turn the machine back on and tap with the rest of the cucumber to gently push the sprouts and spinach through, and then juice the remaining part of the cucumber. Stir the juice, pour into a glass, and drink as soon as possible.
SERVES 1

## MINT REFRESHER

2 fennel stalks with leaves
1/2 cucumber, washed, or
   peeled if not organic
1/2 green apple such as Granny
   Smith or pippin

1 small handful mint
1-inch chunk gingerroot,
   scrubbed, or peeled if old

Cut the produce to fit your juicer's feed tube. Juice all the ingredients and stir. Pour into a glass and drink as soon as possible.
SERVES 1 TO 2

## MAGNESIUM-RICH BLEND

3 to 4 carrots, scrubbed well,
   tops removed, ends trimmed
2 celery ribs, with leaves if
   desired

1/2 small beet, scrubbed well,
   with 1 or 2 leaves
2 to 3 broccoli florets
1/2 lemon, peeled

Cut the produce to fit your juicer's feed tube. Juice all the ingredients and stir. Pour into a glass and drink as soon as possible.
SERVES 1

## HEALTH BOOSTER AND REVITALIZER RECIPES

### BEAUTIFUL-SKIN COCKTAIL

Cucumber and bell pepper are good sources of the trace mineral silicon, which is recommended to strengthen skin, hair, and fingernails along with bones. In studies, silicon has been shown to reduce signs of aging.

1 cucumber, peeled
1 parsnip, peeled
2 to 3 carrots, scrubbed well,
   tops removed, ends trimmed

1/2 lemon, peeled
1/4 green bell pepper, with
   seeds and ribs

Cut the produce to fit your juicer's feed tube. Juice all the ingredients and stir. Pour into a glass and drink as soon as possible.
SERVES 1 TO 2

## CALCIUM-RICH BONE-STRENGTHENING COCKTAIL

Kale and parsley are high in calcium.

1 cucumber, washed, or peeled
   if not organic
1 to 2 medium-to-large kale
   leaves
1 handful parsley

1 celery rib
1/2 lemon, peeled
1-inch chunk gingerroot,
   scrubbed, or peeled if old

Cut the produce to fit your juicer's feed tube. Juice all the ingredients and stir. Pour into a glass and drink as soon as possible.
SERVES 1 TO 2

## PEPPY PARSLEY

1 bunch parsley
2 celery ribs
1 to 2 carrots, scrubbed well,
   tops removed, ends trimmed

1/2 cucumber, washed, or
   peeled if not organic
1/2 lemon, peeled

Cut the produce to fit your juicer's feed tube. Juice all the ingredients and stir. Pour into a glass and drink as soon as possible.
SERVES 1

## THE REVITALIZER

2 tomatoes
1/2 cucumber, washed, or
   peeled if not organic
6 to 8 string beans

1/2 lemon or lime, peeled
Dash of hot sauce

Cut the produce to fit your juicer's feed tube. Juice the produce and stir in the hot sauce. Pour into a glass and drink as soon as possible.

SERVES 1

## WEIGHT-LOSS HELPER

Jerusalem artichokes contain a substance known as inulin that prolongs carbohydrate metabolism, which helps appetite control. It's also been used to improve liver function, which helps weight loss. The key is to sip this juice slowly when you get a craving for high-fat or high-carb foods.

*1 small Jerusalem artichoke (sunchoke), scrubbed well*
*3 to 4 carrots, scrubbed well, tops removed, ends trimmed*

*1/2 small beet, scrubbed well, with 1 or 2 leaves*

Cut the produce to fit your juicer's feed tube. Juice all the ingredients and stir. Pour into a glass and drink as soon as possible.

SERVES 1

## GOOD SLEEP NIGHTCAP

*1 small handful parsley*
*2 romaine lettuce leaves*
*1/2 cucumber, washed, or peeled if not organic*

*3 carrots, scrubbed well, tops removed, ends trimmed*
*1 celery rib*

Bunch up the parsley and roll it in a romaine leaf. Juice the cucumber and turn off the machine. Add the romaine and parsley, turn the machine back on, and tap them through with a carrot. Juice the remaining produce, stir the juice, and drink as soon as possible.

SERVES 1

## MOOD MENDER

Fennel juice has been used as a traditional tonic to help the body release endorphins, the "feel good" peptides, from the brain into the bloodstream. Endorphins help diminish anxiety and fear and generate euphoria.

*3 fennel stalks, including leaves and flowers*
*3 carrots, scrubbed well, tops removed, ends trimmed*

*2 celery ribs*
*1/2 pear*
*1/2-inch chunk gingerroot, scrubbed, or peeled if old*

Cut the produce to fit your juicer's feed tube. Juice all the ingredients and stir. Pour into a glass and drink as soon as possible.
SERVES 1 TO 2

## HEALTHY SINUS SOLUTION

Radish juice is a traditional remedy for opening up the sinuses and supporting the mucous membranes.

*2 vine-ripened tomatoes*
*1/2 cucumber, washed, or peeled if not organic*

*6 radishes, scrubbed*
*1/2 lime, peeled*

Cut the produce to fit your juicer's feed tube. Juice all the ingredients and stir. Pour into a glass and drink as soon as possible.
SERVES 1

## THE IMMUNE SUPPORTER

Studies show that garlic contains a compound that has a natural antibiotic-like effect and is very helpful for the immune system. It is antibacterial, antifungal, antiparasitic, and antiviral, but it must be consumed raw to have this effect.

1 handful watercress
1 turnip, scrubbed, top
    removed, end trimmed
1 to 2 garlic cloves
1/2 green apple such as Granny

Smith or pippin, or 1/2
lemon, peeled
3 carrots, scrubbed well, tops
    removed, ends trimmed

Bunch up the watercress. Cut the produce to fit your juicer's feed tube. Tuck the watercress in the feed tube and push through with the turnip. Juice the remaining ingredients, finishing with one of the carrots. Stir the juice, pour into a glass, and drink as soon as possible.

SERVES 1

## PANCREAS-HELPER COCKTAIL

Brussels sprouts and string bean juice have been used as traditional remedies to help strengthen and support the pancreas. Drink this juice before a meal. (If this juice is too strong, dilute it with a little water.) For the best pancreas support, also avoid refined carbohydrates such as white flour products, sugars of all types, soft drinks, and all sweets.

2 romaine lettuce leaves
1/2 cucumber, washed, or
    peeled if not organic
1 large vine-ripened tomato

8 to 10 string beans
2 Brussels sprouts
1/2 lemon, peeled

Bunch up the romaine leaves. Cut the produce to fit your juicer's feed tube. Tuck the romaine in the feed tube and push through with the cucumber. Juice the remaining ingredients, finishing with some of the tomato. Pour into a glass and drink as soon as possible.

SERVES 1

## HEALTHY-LUNG SOLUTION

Turnip juice has been used as a traditional remedy to strengthen lung tissue.

*1 handful watercress*
*1 small turnip, scrubbed well,*
*    top removed, end trimmed*
*2-inch-thick chunk of jicama,*
*    scrubbed well or peeled*

*2 to 3 carrots, scrubbed*
*    well, tops removed, ends*
*    trimmed*
*1 garlic clove (unpeeled)*
*1/2 lemon, peeled*

Bunch up the watercress. Cut the produce to fit your juicer's feed tube. Tuck the watercress in the feed tube and push through with the turnip. Juice the remaining ingredients, finishing with one of the carrots. Stir the juice, pour into a glass, and drink as soon as possible.

SERVES 1

## ARTHRITIS MENDER

Ginger has anti-inflammatory properties that can help reduce arthritic joint pain and help combat oxidative stress in the joints. Spinach is rich in vitamin K, which helps regulate the inflammatory response.

*1 handful spinach*
*3 to 4 carrots, scrubbed well,*
*    tops removed, ends trimmed*
*2 celery ribs, with leaves*

*2-inch-chunk gingerroot*
*1 lemon, peeled if not*
*    organic*

Cut the produce to fit your juicer's feed tube. Juice remaining ingredients and stir. Pour into a glass and drink as soon as possible.

SERVES 1

## BLOOD-BUILDING TONIC

Dandelion leaves are rich in iron and are good tonics for your blood. They are also rich in vitamin C, which makes iron more absorbable. They are also very cleansing for the blood and liver. But they are quite bitter, so don't expect this juice recipe to taste delicious.

1 cucumber, washed, or peeled          2 celery ribs
   if not organic                                1/2 lemon, peeled if not organic
1 handful dandelion greens

Cut the produce to fit your juicer's feed tube. Start by juicing half the cucumber. Add the dandelion greens, followed by the celery, lemon, and remaining cucumber. Stir the juice and pour into a glass. Drink as soon as possible.

SERVES 1 TO 2

## DIGESTION TONIC

Pear has been used traditionally for weak digestive systems. Drink a glass of this tonic in the morning and evening.

1/2 pear, washed                               1/4 medium jicama, scrubbed
1 cucumber, washed, or peeled             well or peeled if not
   if not organic                                   organic
5 carrots, scrubbed well, tops
   removed, ends trimmed

Cut the pear into sections that will fit your juicer's feed tube. Juice the pear with the cucumber, carrots, and jicama. Stir the juice and pour into a glass. For a weak digestive system or if you have a lung condition, serve this juice at room temperature (chilled is too hard on weak lungs and a compromised intestinal tract); otherwise, serve chilled, if desired.

SERVES 1

## HANGOVER-HELPER COCKTAIL

The liver is adversely affected by overconsumption of alcohol. Tomato juice combined with string bean juice and a dash of hot sauce will help revitalize the liver and improve vitality. Alcohol also is very dehydrating; this juice combination helps hydrate the body quickly.

*2 medium to large vine-ripened tomatoes, washed*
*1/2 organic cucumber*
*6 organic string beans, washed*

*1/4 lime or lemon, washed, or peeled if not organic*
*Dash of hot sauce*

Cut the tomatoes into sections that will fit your juicer's feed tube and cut the cucumber lengthwise in half. Juice the tomatoes, cucumber, string beans, and lime or lemon. Pour the juice into a glass, add the hot sauce, and stir until well mixed. Serve at room temperature or chilled, as desired.

SERVES 1

## SINUS HEALER

Radish juice is a traditional remedy to open sinus cavities and strengthen mucous membranes.

*2 medium vine-ripened tomatoes*
*1 cucumber, washed, or peeled if not organic*

*4 radishes with tops*
*1/2 lime or lemon, washed, or peeled if not organic*

Cut the tomato into sections that will fit your juicer's feed tube. Juice the tomatoes with the cucumber, radishes, and lime or lemon. Stir the juice and pour into a glass. Serve at room temperature or chilled, as desired.

ES 1

## THYROID REVITALIZER

Radish juice has been used as a traditional remedy to promote a healthy thyroid, along with iodine-rich foods such as sea vegetables and cranberries.

*5 carrots, scrubbed well, tops removed, ends trimmed*
*5 to 6 radishes with tops, washed well*
*1/2 lemon, washed, or peeled if not organic*

*1 celery rib with leaves*
*1/2 cucumber, washed, or peeled if not organic*

Juice the carrots, radishes, lemon, celery, and cucumber. Stir the juice and pour into a glass. Serve at room temperature or chilled, as desired.

SERVES 1

## KIDNEY TONIC

Asparagus juice is a traditional remedy to promote healthy kidneys and prostate. Asparagus juice also is a natural diuretic. Juice the stems and use the tips, lightly steamed or grilled, with a meal.

*2 carrots, scrubbed well, green tops removed*
*1 cucumber, washed, or peeled if not organic*

*8 asparagus stems, washed*
*1/2 lemon, peeled if not organic*

Cut the produce to fit your juicer's feed tube. Juice all the ingredients. Stir the juice and pour into a glass. Serve at room temperature or chilled, as desired.

SERVES 1

# Green Smoothies, Blender Drinks, and Shakes

## CHERIE'S GREEN DELIGHT

1/2 English cucumber, washed, or peeled if not organic, and cut into chunks

1 avocado, peeled, seeded, and cut into quarters

1 cup raw spinach

1/2 to 3/4 cup coconut milk

Juice of 1 lime

1 tablespoon green powder of choice (optional)

2 to 3 tablespoons ground almonds (optional)

Combine the cucumber, avocado, spinach, coconut milk, lime juice, and green powder (if desired) in a blender and blend well. Sprinkle the ground almonds on top, if desired.

SERVES 2

## THE HEALTHY NUT

1 cup unsweetened pineapple juice (juice from about 1/4 small pineapple, if making fresh juice)

10 almonds, whole or blanched

1 tablespoon sunflower seeds

1 tablespoon sesame seeds

1 tablespoon flaxseed

1 tablespoon chia seeds (optional)

1 cup chopped parsley

1/2 cup almond, rice, or sesame milk

1/2 teaspoon pure vanilla extract

1 tablespoon protein powder

6 ice cubes

ce the pineapple juice, nuts, and seeds in a bowl, cover, and
overnight at room temperature. Place this nut and seed
re with the juice in the blender and add the parsley, milk,
protein powder, and ice cubes. Blend on high speed

until smooth. This smoothie will be a bit chewy because of the nuts and seeds. It makes a great breakfast.

Tip: To kill molds, when soaking nuts and seeds, add 1/2 teaspoon ascorbic acid to the pineapple juice.

SERVES 2

## GREEN MONKEY SHAKE

1 cup chopped frozen mango
1 cup chopped kale
1/2 cup chopped cucumber, washed, or peeled if not organic

Juice of 1 lime or lemon
4 to 5 ice cubes

Combine all ingredients in a blender and process well, until smooth and creamy. Serve chilled.

SERVES 2

## BERRY GREEN SMOOTHIE

1 cucumber, peeled if not organic
1 cup blueberries, fresh, or thawed if frozen
1/2 cup fresh apple juice
3 to 4 dark chard leaves, chopped

1/2 cup baby spinach
1-inch-chunk gingerroot
Juice of 1/2 lemon, peeled if not organic
1 avocado, peeled, seeded, and cut into chunks

Cut the cucumber into chunks. Place the cucumber, berries, and apple juice in a blender and process until smooth. Chop the greens and ginger and add to the blender along with the lemon juice and avocado. Process until well blended.

SERVES 2

## GREEN POWER PRO

3 kale leaves, chopped
3 chard leaves, chopped
1/2 cup parsley, chopped
1 pear, stems removed, cut into
    chunks

1 banana, peeled and cut into
    chunks
1/2 cup almond, hemp, or
    coconut milk

Combine all ingredients in a blender and process until smooth and creamy. Pour into glasses and serve immediately.
SERVES 2

## THE ISLANDER

1/2 ripe mango, peeled, pitted,
    and cut into chunks
1/2 papaya, peeled, seeded,
    and cut into chunks

1/2 cup coconut milk
1/2 cup baby spinach
6 ice cubes

Place all ingredients in a blender and process until smooth and creamy. Pour into a glass and serve chilled.
SERVES 1

## HEAVY-METAL CLEANSING SHAKE

Cilantro helps detox mercury and other heavy metals.

1 handful of cilantro
1 cup chopped fresh parsley
1/2 cup chopped cucumber,
    washed, or peeled if not
    organic

1 mango, peeled and seeded,
    cut into chunks
1/2 cup fresh apple juice
Juice of 1 lemon

Combine all ingredients in a blender and process until smooth and creamy. Pour into glasses and serve immediately.
SERVES 2

## HAPPY GREEN MORNIN'

1 cucumber, washed, or peeled
   if not organic and chopped
1/2 cup chopped kale

1/2 cup frozen papaya
6 to 8 ice cubes

Combine all ingredients in a blender and process until smooth and creamy. Pour into a glass and serve chilled.

SERVES 1

## COCONUT-ALMOND BREEZE

1 cup chopped mango
1 cup packed baby spinach
3/4 cup almond milk
1/4 cup grated unsweetened
   coconut, lightly packed

2 teaspoons organic lime peel,
   freshly grated
1 teaspoon pure vanilla extract

Combine all ingredients in a blender and process until smooth and creamy. Serve immediately.

SERVES 1 TO 2

## VERY VEGGIE GREEN SMOOTHIE

1 1/4 cups fresh cucumber juice
   (about l large or 2 medium
   cucumbers, peeled if not
   organic)
2 celery ribs with leaves, juiced
1 kale leaf, chopped
1 avocado, peeled, seeded, and
   cut into chunks

1 garlic clove, peeled
Juice of 1 lemon
1/2 cup flat leaf parsley,
   coarsely chopped
2 teaspoons sweet onion, minced
1 teaspoon dried dill weed

Pour the cucumber and celery juices into a blender; add the kale, avocado, garlic, lemon juice, parsley, onion, and dill. Blend on high speed until smooth and creamy; serve immediately, as it does not taste good if it sits.

SERVES 2

## BLUEBERRY-COCONUT HEALTH SHAKE

*1 cup coconut milk*
*1 cup blueberries*
*1 cup packed baby spinach*
*1 tablespoon organic virgin*
*coconut oil*

*1 tablespoon ground flaxseeds*
*1 teaspoon pure vanilla extract*
*1/4 teaspoon almond extract*
*2 to 3 drops stevia*
*6 to 8 ice cubes*

Combine all ingredients except ice in a blender, and process until creamy and smooth. Add ice after the coconut oil is blended so that it won't clump. You may use more or less ice, depending on how cold you like your smoothie.

SERVES 1 TO 2

## LIVER-CLEANSING SMOOTHIE

*1 pear, Bartlett or Asian*
*1 large handful dandelion*
*greens*
*1 cup almond milk*

*Juice of 1/2 lemon, peeled if not*
*organic*
*1/4 cup flaxseeds*
*6 ice cubes (optional)*

Place all ingredients in a blender and process until creamy and smooth.

SERVES 2

## SWEET KALE SHAKE

*1 cucumber, washed, or peeled*
*if not organic*
*1 cup chopped kale*
*1 apple*

*1 avocado, peeled, seeded, and*
*cut into chunks*
*6 ice cubes*

Chop the cucumber, kale, and apple. Place in the blender and process until smooth. Add the avocado and ice, and blend until creamy.

SERVES 2

## SPICY CARROT SHAKE

1 cup carrot juice (about 8
 carrots)
1 apple, cut into chunks

1 cup packed baby spinach
1-inch-chunk gingerroot
6 ice cubes

Place all ingredients in a blender and process until smooth.
Pour into glasses and serve chilled.

SERVES 2

## NUTTY APPLE-BERRY SHAKE

1/2 cup fresh apple juice
1 cup fresh or frozen berries
1/2 cup raw cashews

1 cup chopped chard or kale
6 ice cubes

Pour the apple juice into a blender and add the berries, cashews,
chard, and ice. Blend on high speed until smooth; serve immediately.

SERVES 1

## SIMPLY REFRESHING SHAKE

1/2 cucumber, peeled and cut
 into chunks
1 celery rib, juiced or chopped
 into small pieces
Juice of 1/2 lemon
1/2 teaspoon freshly grated

lemon peel, preferably
 organic
1/2 teaspoon ascorbic acid
 (vitamin C powder)
Nutritional yeast (optional)

Place the cucumber chunks in a freezer bag and freeze them
until solid. Combine the frozen cucumber chunks in a blender
with the celery, lemon juice, lemon peel, and ascorbic acid.
Blend on high speed until smooth, sprinkle with nutritional
yeast as desired, and serve immediately.

SERVES 1

## GREEN COCONUT SHAKE

1 cup coconut milk

1 cup packed baby spinach

1 tablespoon virgin coconut oil

1 tablespoon ground flaxseeds

1 teaspoon pure vanilla extract

1/4 teaspoon almond extract

1/4 teaspoon stevia powder

8 to 10 ice cubes

Place all the ingredients but the ice in a blender and process at high speed until well combined. Add the ice after the coconut oil is blended so that it won't clump. You may use more or less ice, depending on how cold you like your smoothie.

SERVES 1 TO 2

## TOMATO WITH A TWIST

2 tomatoes, cut into chunks

1 cup tomato juice (2 to 3 medium tomatoes, juiced)

1/2 lemon, juiced

1 teaspoon freshly grated lemon peel, preferably organic

6 fresh basil leaves, rinsed

Place the tomato chunks in a freezer bag and freeze them until solid. Pour the tomato juice into a blender and add the frozen tomato chunks, lemon juice, lemon peel, and basil. Blend on high speed until smooth, and serve immediately.

SERVES 1

## ICY SPICY TOMATO

2 tomatoes, cut into chunks

1 cup fresh carrot juice (about 5 to 7 carrots, juiced)

1/2 lemon, juiced, peeled if using a juice machine

2 tablespoons rinsed chopped cilantro

1/4 teaspoon sea salt

1/4 teaspoon ground cumin

1/4 small jalapeño, chopped, or to taste

3 radishes, washed and chopped

Place the tomato chunks in a freezer bag and freeze them until solid. Pour the carrot and lemon juices into a blender and add the frozen tomato chunks, cilantro, salt, cumin, jalapeño, and radishes. Blend on high speed until smooth and serve immediately.
SERVES 1

## SALSA SHAKE

1 cup chopped tomato
1 cup fresh cucumber juice (1/2 cucumber, peeled if not organic, and juiced) or 1/2 cucumber, peeled, cut into chunks, and frozen
1 lemon, juiced

1/2 teaspoon freshly grated lemon peel, preferably organic
2 daikon radishes, washed (optional)
Dash cayenne pepper

Place the tomato chunks (and the cucumber chunks if freezing) in a freezer bag and freeze them until solid. Pour the cucumber juice or place the frozen cucumber chunks and the lemon juice in a blender and add the frozen tomato chunks, lemon peel, daikon radishes, if using, and cayenne. Blend on high speed until smooth, and serve immediately.
SERVES 1 TO 2

## RAW SOUPS

## ENERGY SOUP

2 to 3 carrots, scrubbed, tops removed, ends trimmed
2 to 3 celery ribs
1/2 cucumber, washed, or peeled if not organic
1/2 lemon, peeled and seeded
Handful of parsley

1- to 2-inch chunk gingerroot, peeled
1 avocado, peeled, seeded, and cut into quarters
Grated zucchini, fresh corn, or crunchy sprouts such as pea, lentil, and bean, for garnish

Juice the carrots, celery, cucumber, lemon, parsley, and ginger-root. Pour the juice into a blender and add the avocado. Blend until smooth. Pour into bowls and serve immediately. You may garnish with any of the optional additions for a crunchy topper.

SERVES 2

## YUMMY BROCCOLI SOUP

1 cup vegetable stock
1 to 2 cups chopped broccoli
1/2 onion, chopped
1 red or yellow bell pepper, chopped
1 to 2 celery ribs, chopped

1 avocado, peeled, seeded, and cut into quarters
Bragg Liquid Aminos or sea salt
Cumin or grated ginger
Lemon (optional)

Gently warm the vegetable stock, keeping the temperature at or below 118°F. Add the broccoli and onion and warm for 5 minutes. Turn off the heat. Add the bell pepper and celery and allow to sit for an additional 5 minutes.

Puree the vegetable broth mixture in a blender until smooth. Add the avocado and blend until smooth.

Add the Bragg Liquid Aminos or sea salt to taste. If using cumin, add it and blend.

If using grated ginger, add to the soup and stir in.

A squeeze of lemon is nice. Add as desired.

SERVES 2

## SPICY YAM BISQUE

1 cup yam juice
1 cup sesame, almond, or rice milk
1/4 cup chopped red onion
1 avocado, peeled, seeded, and cut into chunks

1 teaspoon nutmeg
1/4 teaspoon cinnamon
1/4 teaspoon ground allspice
1/4 teaspoon ground mace
1/4 teaspoon cardamom

Juice 1 yam or enough to give you 1 cup of juice. Let it sit until the starch settles to the bottom of the measuring cup. This should take about an hour. Pour the clear juice into a blender. Do not use the starchy portion, as this will make the soup gritty; discard.

Add the milk of choice to the blender. Add the onion and avocado and blend until smooth. Add the spices and blend.

SERVES 2

## SPINACH-AVOCADO SOUP

1 avocado, peeled, seeded, and cut into chunks
1 cucumber, peeled, cut into chunks
1 cup spinach
1 small jalapeño, seeded
Juice of 1/2 to 1 lemon

1/2 cup water
1 to 2 cloves garlic
1 tablespoon cilantro
1 tablespoon fresh parsley
1/4 purple onion, finely chopped, for garnish

Place the avocado, cucumber, spinach, jalapeño, lemon juice, water, garlic, cilantro, and parsley in a blender or food processor and puree until smooth. Pour into a bowl and add the chopped onion, or any other chopped vegetables or herbs, as a garnish.

SERVES 2

## CREAMY TOMATO SOUP

1/2 large or 1 small avocado, peeled, seeded, and cut into chunks
1 to 2 vine-ripened tomatoes
2 tablespoons chopped sweet red bell pepper

1/4 carrot, chopped into small pieces
3/4 cup sesame or almond milk

Combine all ingredients in a blender and blend well. Pour into bowls.

SERVES 2

## SUMMER CORN CHOWDER

2 cups fresh or frozen corn
    kernels (about 2 large ears)
1 cup almond milk
1 avocado, peeled, seeded, and
    cut into chunks
1/4 red bell pepper, cut into
    chunks

2 teaspoons chopped onion
1/2 teaspoon ground cumin
1/2 teaspoon sea salt
1 tablespoon each chopped
    parsley and minced red
    bell pepper, for garnish
    (optional)

In a blender, combine the corn, almond milk, avocado, bell pepper, onion, cumin, and salt. Blend well. Pour into bowls and garnish with parsley and red pepper.

SERVES 2

## MINTY CUCUMBER SOUP

1 cucumber, peeled and cut
    into chunks
1 avocado, peeled, seeded, and
    cut into chunks

1/4 cup chopped fresh mint

Combine the cucumber, avocado, and mint in a blender and blend well. Pour into a bowl.

SERVES 1

## GARDEN TOMATO SOUP

3 small or 2 medium tomatoes
2 green onions (about 2 inches
    of tips and greens), chopped
1/2 green pepper, chopped

1 cup vegetable broth
1 avocado, peeled, seeded, and
    cut into quarters
1 teaspoon sea salt

Combine all the ingredients in a blender and blend well. Pour into bowls.

SERVES 2

## FRENCH TOMATO-BASIL SOUP

6 medium tomatoes, cut into
    quarters
1/2 lemon, peeled, seeded, and
    cut into chunks
1 avocado, peeled, seeded, and
    cut into quarters

2 tablespoons chopped fresh
    basil
1 tablespoon chopped onion
1 small garlic clove
Basil leaves, for garnish

In a blender, blend the tomatoes until chunky. Add the lemon, avocado, chopped basil, onion, and garlic. Blend well. Pour into bowls and garnish with fresh basil leaves.

SERVES 2

## HEARTY KALE SOUP

3 large kale leaves
3 celery ribs
1/2 lemon, peeled

1 avocado, peeled, seeded, and
    cut into quarters
1 cup spinach leaves

Juice the kale, celery, and lemon. Pour into a blender, add the avocado and spinach, and blend well. Pour into bowls and serve.

SERVES 2

## VEGETABLE HARVEST SOUP

2 cups water or vegetable
    broth
1 cup chopped green beans
1 cup chopped asparagus
2 carrots, chopped
2 celery ribs, chopped

1/2 onion, chopped
Pinch of mace
1 teaspoon sea salt
1 tablespoon chopped parsley,
    for garnish

Pour the water or vegetable broth into a soup pot. Add the vegetables and gently warm for about 10 minutes, or until the vegetables are just slightly tender. Pour the soup into a blender, add

the mace and sea salt, and blend well. Pour into bowls and garnish with parsley.
SERVES 2

## SPINACH POWER SOUP

1 avocado, peeled, seeded, and
    cut into quarters
1/2 cup water
1 cucumber, peeled and cut
    into chunks
1 green onion, chopped
1/4 red bell pepper,
    chopped

1 clove garlic, chopped
1/2 teaspoon sea salt
1 cup spinach, packed
Raw pumpkin seeds, for
    garnish

Combine the avocado and water in a blender and blend well. Add the cucumber, green onion, bell pepper, garlic, and salt. Blend well. Add the spinach and blend well. Pour into bowls. Garnish with pumpkin seeds.
SERVES 2

## ZIPPY ASPARAGUS SOUP

10 asparagus stalks, chopped
4 tomatoes, cut into chunks
1/4 cup water
1/4 cup chopped fresh parsley
1/4 cup chopped onion
1/2 red bell pepper, chopped
3 to 4 sun-dried tomatoes

2 cloves garlic
1/2 teaspoon sea salt or Bragg
    Liquid Aminos
1 avocado, peeled, seeded, and
    cut into quarters
1/2 lemon (cut into quarters)

Combine the asparagus, tomatoes, water, parsley, onion, bell pepper, sun-dried tomatoes, garlic, and salt or Bragg Liquid Aminos in a blender and blend well. Add the avocado and blend well. Pour into bowls and add a squeeze of lemon to each bowl.
SERVES 2

## REFRESHING TOMATILLO-CUCUMBER SOUP

1 cucumber, peeled and cut
    into chunks
2 tomatillos
1 lime, peeled, seeded, and cut
    into chunks
2 cups fresh baby spinach,
    loosely packed

1/2 cup almond milk
1 avocado, peeled, seeded, and
    cut into quarters
4 to 6 ice cubes

Combine the cucumber, tomatillos, lime, spinach, and almond milk in a blender and blend well. Add the avocado and ice cubes and blend well. Pour into bowls.

SERVES 2


## CREAMY CAULIFLOWER SOUP

1/2 onion, chopped
3 celery ribs, chopped
1 head cauliflower, chopped
1 tablespoon virgin coconut oil

1 cup almond milk
1/2 teaspoon sea salt
Pepper (optional)

Lightly steam the onion, celery, and cauliflower for about 5 minutes or until just tender. Combine in a blender with the coconut oil, almond milk, salt, and pepper to taste. Blend well. Pour into bowls.

SERVES 2


## ZIPPY TOMATO SOUP

2 radishes, scrubbed
2 celery ribs
1/2 lemon, peeled
2 tomatoes, chopped
1 garlic clove, peeled
1 to 2 pickled umebushi plums,
    seeds removed

1/2 teaspoon freshly grated
    lemon peel, preferably
    organic
Dash of cayenne pepper
4 to 6 ice cubes

Juice the radishes, celery, and lemon. Pour the juice into a blender and add the tomatoes, garlic, plums, lemon peel, cayenne, and ice. Blend on high speed until smooth, pour into bowls, and serve immediately.

SERVES 1 TO 2

## CREAMY TOMATO COOLER

2 cups washed, chopped
   tomatoes
1 avocado, chopped
1/2 cup almond or sesame milk
1/2 teaspoon freshly grated
   lemon peel, preferably
   organic

1/2 teaspoon balsamic vinegar
1/2 lemon, juiced
Dash of cayenne pepper
   (optional)

Place the chopped tomato in a freezer bag and freeze until solid. Combine the tomato, avocado, milk, lemon peel, balsamic vinegar, lemon juice, and cayenne as desired in a blender. Blend on high speed until smooth and serve immediately.

SERVES 1 TO 2

## CARROT-TOMATO COOLER

3 medium tomatoes, cut into
   chunks
1 1/2 cups fresh carrot juice ·
   (about 6 large carrots)
1 tablespoon balsamic vinegar
   or fresh lemon juice

2 teaspoons tamari or Bragg
   Liquid Aminos
1 garlic clove, peeled
Finely chopped cilantro or
   parsley, for garnish

Place the tomato chunks in a freezer bag and freeze until solid. Pour the carrot juice, balsamic vinegar or lemon juice, and tamari or Bragg Liquid Aminos into a blender and add the tomato chunks and garlic; blend on high speed until smooth. Garnish as desired and serve immediately.

SERVES 2

## CUCUMBER-AVOCADO SOUP

1 1/4 cups fresh cucumber juice
    (about l large or 2 medium
    cucumbers, peeled if not
    organic, juiced)
2 celery ribs, juiced
1 avocado, peeled, seeded, and
    cut into quarters

1 garlic clove, peeled
1/2 cup almond milk
1/2 cup coarsely chopped
    parsley
2 teaspoons chopped onion
1 teaspoon dried dill weed

Pour the cucumber and celery juices into a blender and add the avocado, garlic, milk, parsley, onion, and dill. Blend on high speed until smooth and serve immediately. This soup is not good if it sits.

SERVES 2

## CREAMY RED PEPPER SOUP

3 large red bell peppers
6 garlic cloves, peeled
1 cup almond milk
1 tablespoon balsamic vinegar
2 teaspoons tamari or Bragg
    Liquid Aminos

6 fresh basil leaves, rinsed
Chopped fresh basil, for
    garnish (optional)

Lightly steam the peppers and garlic for about 5 minutes or just until tender. Cut the peppers into chunks. Pour the milk into a blender and add the peppers, garlic, balsamic vinegar, tamari or Bragg Liquid Aminos, and basil leaves. Blend on high speed until smooth. Pour into bowls and garnish with chopped fresh basil, as desired. Serve immediately.

SERVES 1 TO 2

## CUCUMBER-MINT SOUP

*1 cup almond milk*
*2 cups peeled, diced cucumber*
*1/4 cup chopped scallions*
*1/2 teaspoon sea salt*

*6 mint leaves*
*1 garlic clove, peeled and*
   *minced*

Combine the milk with the cucumber, scallions, salt, mint, and garlic in a blender and process on high speed until smooth. Pour into bowls and serve immediately.

SERVES 2

# Resources Guide

Sign up for the Juice Lady's free *Juice Newsletter* at JuiceLady Cherie.com.

## CHERIE'S WEBSITE

JuiceLadyCherie.com—information on juicing and weight loss

## THE JUICE LADY'S HEALTH AND WELLNESS JUICE CLEANSE RETREATS

I invite you to join us for a week that can change your life! Our retreats offer gourmet organic raw foods with a three-day juice fast midweek. We offer interesting, informative classes for detoxification of body, soul, and spirit in a beautiful, peaceful setting where you can experience healing and restoration. For more information, a brochure, and dates for the retreats, call 866-8GETWEL (866-843-8935).

## SCHEDULE A NUTRITION CONSULTATION WITH THE JUICE LADY

Call 866-8GETWEL (866-843-8935).

## BOOK THE JUICE LADY TO SPEAK FOR YOUR ORGANIZATION

Call 866-8GETWEL (866-843-8935).

## OTHER BOOKS BY CHERIE AND JOHN CALBOM

These books can be ordered at JuiceLadyCherie.com:

Cherie Calbom, *The Juice Lady's Big Book of Juices and Green Smoothies* (Siloam)

Cherie Calbom, *The Juice Lady's Weekend Weight-Loss Diet* (Charisma)

Cherie Calbom, *The Juice Lady's Living Foods Revolution* (Charisma)

Cherie Calbom, *The Juice Lady's Turbo Diet* (Siloam)

Cherie Calbom, *The Juice Lady's Guide to Juicing for Health* (Avery)

Cherie Calbom and John Calbom, *Sleep Away the Pounds* (Wellness Central)

Cherie Calbom, *The Wrinkle Cleanse* (Avery)

Cherie Calbom and John Calbom, *The Coconut Diet* (Wellness Central)

Cherie Calbom, John Calbom, and Michael Mahaffey, *The Complete Cancer Cleanse* (Thomas Nelson)

Cherie Calbom, *The Ultimate Smoothie Book* (Wellness Central)

## JUICERS

Find out about the best juicers recommended by Cherie. Call 866-8GETWEL (866-843-8935), or visit JuiceLadyCherie.com.

## DEHYDRATORS

Find out about the best dehydrators recommended by Cherie. Call 866-8GETWEL (866-843-8935), or visit JuiceLadyCherie.com.

## LYMPHASIZER

To view the swing machine (lymphasizer), visit JuiceLadyCherie
.com, or call 866-8GETWEL (866-843-8935) for more information.

## VEGGIE POWDERS

To purchase or get information on Barley Max, Carrot Juice
Max, and Beet Max powders, go to JuiceLadyCherie.com, or
call 866-8GETWEL (866-843-8935). (These powders are ideal
for when you travel or when you can't get juice.)

## VIRGIN COCONUT OIL

For more information on virgin coconut oil, go to JuiceLady
Cherie.com or GoCoconuts.com, or call 866-8GETWEL
(866-843-8935). To save money, order larger sizes such as gallons or quarts, which you won't typically find in the stores.

## SUPPLEMENTS

For multivitamins by Thorne Research, call 866-8GETWEL
(866-843-8935).

Digestive enzymes Ness Formula #4 and #16 are excellent
to aid digestion. Taken between meals, they help clean up
undigested proteins. With the addition of enzymes, you
should notice that your hair and nails grow better. Call
866-8GETWEL (866-843-8935).

For Magnesium citrate or Magnesium Citramate (as magnesium citrate-malate and malic acid) by Thorne Research, call
866-8GETWEL (866-843-8935).

For vitamin C with bioflavonoids or Buffered C Powder (contains ascorbic acid, calcium, magnesium, and potassium) by
Thorne Research or Allergy Research, call 866-8GETWEL
(866-843-8935).

For vitamin D3 (1,000 or 5,000 milligrams) by Thorne Research, call 866-8GETWEL (866-843-8935).

## COLON-CLEANSE PRODUCTS

Call 866-8GETWEL (866-843-8935) for more information on Cherie's fiber recommendations:
Medibulk by Thorne (psyllium powder, prune powder, apple pectin)

### Colon-Cleanse Kit

After years of eating standard food, it's quite common to build up a layer of mucoid plaque—hardened mucus-like material and food residue that can coat the gastrointestinal tract. Nutrients are absorbed through the intestinal wall. The plaque hinders our ability to absorb nutrients, which can lead to numerous health problems. This colon-cleanse kit contains products that can pull the plaque from your intestinal wall and carry it out of your system—Digestive Stimulator, Toxin Absorber, glass shaker jar, and user guide and dosage calendar. Specify ginger or peppermint flavor. For more information, go to JuiceLadyCherie.com.

## INTERNAL CLEANSING KIT

The complete and comprehensive internal cleansing kit contains eighteen items for a twenty-one-day cleanse program, You get a free colon-cleanse kit, along with Liver-Gallbladder Rejuvenator, Friendly Bacteria Replenisher, Parasite Cleanser, Lung Rejuvenator, Kidney and Bladder Rejuvenator, Blood and Skin Rejuvenator, and Lymph Rejuvenator, along with a glass shaker jar and user guide and dosage calendar. Specify ginger or peppermint flavor. Cost: $279, less 5 percent discount.
You may order cleansing products and get the 10 percent discount by calling 866-8GETWEL (866-843-8935). If you want

to read more about the cleansing kits, go to my website, JuiceLadyCherie.com. You will need to order via the toll-free number to get the discount; just mention my special book discount price.

### *CANDIDA ALBICANS* CLEANSE PRODUCTS

For the Total Body Internal Cleanse Kit, visit JuiceLadyCherie .com, or call 866-8GETWEL (866-843-8935).

### HEAVY-METAL CLEANSE PRODUCTS

MetalloClear is designed to help patients stay healthy by providing specialized support for heavy-metal metabolism.
Heavy Metal Support by Thorne replaces important minerals and other nutrients lost during metal chelating.

### KIDNEY CLEANSE

For Kidney and Bladder Rejuvenator, visit JuiceLadyCherie.com, or call 866-8GETWEL (866-843-8935).

### LIVER/GALLBLADDER-CLEANSE PRODUCTS

Detox Nutrients Packet (Liver Cleanse)
Complete supplement "take-anywhere" packets for detoxification support. Order at JuiceLadyCherie.com.
For Chinese herbal tinctures (four-part kit) to use with Cherie's Liver Detox Program, call 866-8GETWEL (866-843-8935).

### LUNG REJUVENATOR

Visit JuiceLadyCherie.com, or call 866-8GETWEL (866-843-8935).

### LYMPH REJUVENATOR

Visit JuiceLadyCherie.com, or call 866-8GETWEL (866-843-8935).

## PARASITE-CLEANSE PRODUCTS

For Large Para Cleanser 1 and 2 and Small Para Cleanser, visit JuiceLadyCherie.com.

For Total Body Internal Cleanse Kit (includes Para Cleanse Kit and a free colon cleanse kit), visit JuiceLadyCherie.com, or call 866-8GETWEL (866-843-8935).

## SKIN AND BLOOD REJUVENATOR

Visit JuiceLadyCherie.com, or call 866-8GETWEL (866-843-8935).

## SLEEP DISORDERS

Testing neurotransmitters is the best way to determine if you have a depletion in brain chemicals that could be causing sleep problems. Testing can be completed whether you are taking medications or not. You can determine if your neurotransmitters are out of balance by taking the Brain Wellness Programs Self Test. Just go to Neurogistics.com and click "Get Started." Use the practitioner code SLEEP (all caps). You can order the program, which includes an in-home urine test that will yield a report on your neurotransmitter levels. You'll be given a customized protocol with guidelines for the right amino acids for you to take to help correct your imbalances. Or you can call 866-8GETWEL (866-843-8935) for more information.

# References

### CHAPTER ONE

Anderson, Rich. *The Liver: Cleansing and Rejuvenating the Vital Organ.* Medford, OR: Christobe Publishing, 1999.

Baker, Arthur M. "Raw fresh produce vs. cooked food." http://www.rawfoodlife.com.

BBC News online. "Organic food 'proven' healthier." January 3, 2000. http://news.bbc.co.uk/2/hi/science/nature.

Calbom, Cherie, and John Calbom. *The Coconut Diet.* New York: Warner, 2005.

Calbom, Cherie, John Calbom, and Michael Mahaffey. *The Complete Cancer Cleanse.* Nashville, TN: Thomas Nelson, 2003.

Cornforth, Tracee. "Environmental toxins and reproductive health." http://pms.about.com/b/2009/07/09/environmental-toxins-and-reproductive-health.htm.

Cross, C. E., et al. "Oxygen radicals and human diseases." *Annals of Internal Medicine* 107 (1987): 526.

Harman, D. "Free radical theory of aging: Role of free radicals in the origination and evolution of life, aging, and disease processes." *Free Radicals, Aging, and Degenerative Diseases,* edited by J. E. Johnson, 3–50. New York: Alan R. Liss, 1986.

Koebnick, Corinna, et al. "Long-term consumption of a raw food diet is associated with favorable serum LDL cholesterol and triglycerides but also with elevated plasma homocysteine and low serum HDL cholesterol in humans." *Journal of Nutrition* 122, no. 4 (April 1992): 924–30.

Mayeda, Andrew. "Test finds MPs' bodies full of toxins." *Vancouver Sun* online, January 4, 2007. http://www.canada.com/vancouversun/news/story.html?id=7ccc417c-e082-40ac-a203-303e288c2cb9&k=19093.

Mercola, Joseph. "Scientists warn—dangerous chemical found in plastic." August 7, 2007. http://articles.mercola.com/sites/articles/archive/2007/08/07/scientists-warn-of-the-dangers-of-a-chemical-found-in-plastic.aspx.

———. "The toxic import from China hidden in this everyday beverage…" October 11, 2011. http://articles.mercola.com/sites/articles/archive/2011/10/11/dr-bill-osmunson-on-fluoride.aspx.

———. "The truth about tap water." August 6, 2007. http://articles.mercola.com/sites/articles/archive/2007/08/06/the-truth-about-tap-water.aspx.

———. "Why did the Russians ban an appliance found in 90% of American homes?" May 18, 2010. http://articles.mercola.com/sites/articles/archive/2010/05/18/microwave-hazards.aspx.

Schneider, Andrew. "That buttery aroma might be toxic, too." *Seattle Post-Intelligencer*, August 30, 2007.

Sinatra, Stephen, MD. "Toxin exposure in infancy affects health for a lifetime." *Heart, Health, and Nutrition* (newsletter), August 2007, 2–4.

U.S. Centers for Disease Control and Prevention. "National report on human exposure to environmental chemicals." July 21, 2005. http://www.cdc.gov/media/pressrel/r050721.htm.

U.S. Environmental Protection Agency. "Endocrine disruptor screening program (EDSP)." 1996. http://www.epa.gov/endo.

U.S. Food and Drug Administration, Center for Biologics Evaluation and Research. "Thimerosal in vaccines." http://www.fda.gov/cber/vaccine/thimerosal.htm.

Vandenberg, Laura N., Russ Hauser, Michele Marcus, Nicolas Olea, and Wade V. Welshons. "Human exposure to bisphenol A (BPA)." *Human Toxicology* 25 (July 2007).


CHAPTER TWO

Appel, L. J., T. J. Moore, E. Obarzanek, et al. "A clinical trial of the effects of dietary patterns on blood pressure." DASH Collaborative Research Group. *New England Journal of Medicine* 336 (1997): 1117–24.

"Aspartame and dieting." *Nutrition Week* 27, no. 23 (June 13, 1997); *International Journal of Obesity* 21, no. 1 (January 1997): 37–42.

Brown, L., E. B. Rimm, J. M. Seddon, et al. "A prospective study of carotenoid intake and risk of cataract extraction in U.S. men." *American Journal of Clinical Nutrition* 70 (1999): 517–24.

Calbom, Cherie, MS. *The Juice Lady's Guide to Juicing for Health.* New York: Avery, 1999.

———. *The Juice Lady's Juicing for High-Level Wellness and Vibrant Good Looks.* New York: Three Rivers Press, 1999.

"Cancer and tomatoes." *Nutrition Week* 7 (December 15, 1995); *Journal of the National Cancer Institute* (December 6, 1995).

Center for Nutrition Policy and Promotion. "2005 dietary guidelines for Americans." U.S. Department of Agriculture.

Cheney, G., et al. "Anti-peptic ulcer dietary factor (vitamin 'U') in the treatment of peptic ulcers." *Journal of the American Dietetic Association* 25 (1950): 668–72.

Cho, E., J. M. Seddon, B. Rosner, W. C. Willett, and S. E. Hankinson. "Prospective study of intake of fruits, vegetables, vitamins, and carotenoids and risk of age-related maculopathy." *Archives of Ophthalmology* 122 (2004): 883–92.

Djousse, L., D. K. Arnett, H. Coon, M. A. Province, L. L. Moore, and R. C. Ellison. "Fruit and vegetable consumption and LDL cholesterol: The National Heart, Lung, and Blood Institute Family Heart Study." *American Journal of Clinical Nutrition* 79 (2004): 213–17.

Environmental Working Group. *Food News: Shopper's Guide.* 5th edition. Data are from the USFDA between 2000 and 2005. http://www.foodnews.org/index.php.

FoodNavigator-USA.com. "Pure juices can reduce disease risk." http://www.foodnavigator-usa.com.

"GMO corn causes liver, kidney problems in rats: Study." Reuters.com. March 13, 2007. http://www.reuters.com/article/2007/03/13/us-monsanto-greenpeace-idUSL1346840020070313.

Gupta, Chris. "Nutrition and cooking/freezing." September 24, 2005. http://www.newmediaexplorer.org/chris/2003/10/18/nutrition_and_cookingfreezing.htm.

Harvard School of Public Health. "Healthy eating plate and healthy eating pyramid." http://www.hsph.harvard.edu/nutritionsource/pyramid.

Hung, H. C., K. J. Joshipura, R. Jiang, et al. "Fruit and vegetable intake and risk of major chronic disease." *Journal of National Cancer Institute* 96 (2004): 1577–84.

"Hungary hopeful it can keep its GMO ban." Reuters.com. http://www.reuters.com/article/2007/02/05/us-gmo-hungary-eu-idUSL0533046520070205.

Kjeldsen-Kragh, J., et al. "Controlled trial of fasting and one year vegetarian diet in rheumatoid arthritis." *Lancet* 338 (October 12, 1991): 899–902.

Krinsky, N. I., J. T. Landrum, and R. A. Bone. "Biologic mechanisms of the protective role of lutein and zeaxanthin in the eye." *Annual Review of Nutrition* 23 (2003): 171–201.

Mayo Clinic Staff. "Dry macular degeneration." August 2006. http://www.mayoclinic.com/health/macular-degeneration/DS00284.

Mercola, Joseph. "Genetically modified foods—what to know before you eat them." August 2, 2007. http://articles.mercola .com/sites/articles/archive/2007/08/02/genetically-modified -organisms-are-a-looming-threat.aspx.

———. "How do you know if your food is genetically modified?" January 24, 2004. http://www.mercola.com/2004/jan/24/gm _foods.htm.

———. "Liquid candy becoming the preferred breakfast drink." February 1, 2007. http://articles.mercola.com/sites/articles/ archive/2007/02/01/liquid-candy-becoming-the-preferred -breakfast-drink.aspx.

Moeller, S. M., A. Taylor, K. L. Tucker, et al. "Overall adherence to the dietary guidelines for Americans is associated with reduced prevalence of early age-related nuclear lens opacities in women." *Journal of Nutrition* 134 (2004): 1812–19.

Morse, Robert, ND. *The Detox Miracle Sourcebook*. Prescott, AZ: Holm Press, 2004.

Poulter, Sean. "Cancer row over GM foods as study says it did THIS to rats…and can cause organ damage and early death in humans." September 19, 2012. http://www.dailymail .co.uk/sciencetech/article-2205509/Cancer-row-GM-foods -French-study-claims-did-THIS-rats–cause-organ-damage -early-death-humans.html.

Séralini, Gilles-Eric, et al. "New analysis of a rat feeding study with a genetically modified maize reveals signs of hepatorenal toxicity." *Archives of Environmental Contamination and Toxicology* (March 14, 2007). http://www.springerlink.com/content/ 02648wu132m07804/?p=a4782763081842a38c67449a8b48e 6d3&pi=6.

Tortora, Gerard J., and Sandra R. Grabowski. *Introduction to the Human Body: The Essentials of Anatomy and Physiology*. 6th edition. Hoboken, NJ: John Wiley & Sons, 2004.

Tsang, Gloria, RD. "Fiber 101: soluble fiber vs insoluble fiber." Healthcastle.com. November 2005. http://www.healthcastle .com/fiber-solubleinsoluble.shtml.

U.S. Centers for Disease Control and Prevention. "Fruits and vegetables." http://www.cdc.gov/nutrition/everyone/fruitsveg etables/index.html.

Vainio, H., and F. Bianchini. *IARC Handbooks of Cancer Prevention: Fruit and Vegetables*. Vol. 8. Lyon, France: IARC, 2003.

Young, Emma. "GM pea causes allergic damage in mice." New Scientist.com. November 21, 2005. http://www.newscientist .com/article/dn8347-gm-pea-causes-allergic-damage-in-mice .html.


## CHAPTER THREE

"Alkalinity." www.snyderhealth.com/alkalinity.htm.

Calbom, Cherie, MS. *The Juice Lady's Guide to Juicing for Health*. New York: Avery, 1999.

———. *The Juice Lady's Juicing for High-Level Wellness and Vibrant Good Looks*. New York: Three Rivers Press, 1999.

Colbert, Don, MD. *Toxic Relief: Restore Health and Energy Through Fasting and Detoxification*. Lake Mary, FL: Siloam, 2003.

Floyd, Ronnie W. *The Power of Prayer and Fasting: 10 Secrets of Spiritual Strength*. Nashville, TN: Broadman & Holman, 1997.

Fourest-Fontecave, S., U. Adamson, P. E. Lins, B. Ekblom, C. Sandahl, and L. Strand. "Mental alertness in response to hypoglycaemia in normal man: The effect of 12 hours and 72 hours of fasting." *NCBI PubMed/Diabète et métabolisme* 13, no. 4 (July–August 1987): 405–10. http://www.ncbi.nlm .nih.gov/entrez/query.fcgi?cmd=Retrieve&db=PubMed&list _uids=3315761&dopt=Abstract.

Lagerquist, Ron. *Fasting to Freedom: A Revolution of Body and Spirit*. Revised edition. Sunderland, ON: Renewed Health, 2003.

———. http://www.freedomyou.com.

Mercola, Joseph. http://www.mercola.com.

Morse, Robert, ND. *The Detox Miracle Sourcebook*. Prescott, AZ: Holm Press, 2004.

Seewald, Peter, ed. *Wisdom of the Monastery*. Old Saybrook, CT: Konecky & Konecky, 2003.

Shelton, H. M. *Fasting Can Save Your Life*. Bridgeport, CT: American Natural Hygiene Society, 1991.


CHAPTER FOUR

Anderson, Richard. *The Liver: Cleansing and Rejuvenating the Vital Organ*. Medford, OR: Christobe Publishing, 1999.

Calbom, Cherie, and John Calbom. *The Coconut Diet*. New York: Warner, 2005.

Calbom, Cherie, John Calbom, and Michael Mahaffey. *The Complete Cancer Cleanse*. Nashville, TN: Thomas Nelson, 2003.

Colbert, Don, MD. *Toxic Relief: Restore Health and Energy Through Fasting and Detoxification*. Lake Mary, FL: Siloam, 2003.

Lerner, Ben, DC. "Things you need to know about toxicity." eNewsletter, no. 14, March 6, 2007. Maximizedliving@ ecommunications.ca.

———. "While you were sleeping." eNewsletter, no. 10, February 7, 2007. Maximizedliving@ecommunications.ca.

Mercola, Joseph. "The new epidemic sweeping across America (and it's not a disease)." http://articles.mercola.com/sites/articles/archive/2011/10/26/prescription-drugs-number-one-cause-preventable-death-in-us.aspx.

Morse, Robert, ND. *The Detox Miracle Sourcebook*. Prescott, AZ: Holm Press, 2004.

Null, G., C. Dean, M. Feldman, D. Rasio, and D. Smith. "Death by medicine." Life Extension Foundation, March 2004. http://www.webdc.com/pdfs/deathbymedicine.pdf.

Saxon, V. "Chronic fatigue syndrome." Valerie Saxon's Silver Creek Labs, n.d.

Tortora, G., and S. Grabowski. *Introduction to the Human Body: The Essentials of Anatomy and Physiology*. Hoboken, NJ: John Wiley & Sons, 2004.

U.S. Environmental Protection Agency. "Endocrine disruptor screening program (EDSP)." 1996. http://www.epa.gov/scipoly/oscpendo/pubs/edspoverview/background.htm.

Watson, Brenda. *Renew Your Life*. Clearwater, FL: Renew Life Press, 2002.

Whitney, M. T. "Prescription drug deaths skyrocket 68 percent over five years as Americans swallow more pills." February 22, 2007. http://www.naturalnews.com/021635_prescription_drug_deaths_the_FDA.html.

## CHAPTER FIVE

Calbom, Cherie, and John Calbom. *The Coconut Diet*. New York: Warner, 2005.

Calbom, Cherie, John Calbom, and Michael Mahaffey. *The Complete Cancer Cleanse*. Nashville, TN: Thomas Nelson, 2003.

Chao, A., M. J. Thun, C. J. Connell, M. L. McCullough, E. J. Jacobs, W. D. Flanders, C. Rodriguez, R. Sinha, and E. E. Calle. "Meat consumption and risk of colorectal cancer." *Journal of the American Medical Association* 293 (2005): 172–82. http://www.ncbi.nlm.nih.gov/entrez/query.fcgi?cmd=Retrieve&db=pubmed&dopt=Abstract&list_uids=15644544.

Colbert, Don, MD. *Toxic Relief: Restore Health and Energy Through Fasting and Detoxification*. Lake Mary, FL: Siloam, 2003.

Health-Science.com. "Intestinal ecology." http://www.health-science.com/intestinal_health.html.

Jensen, B., DC. *Tissue Cleansing Through Bowel Management*. Escondido, CA: Bernard Jensen Press, 1981.

MedicineWorld.org. "Colon cancer statistics." http://medicineworld.org/cancer/colon/stat.html.

Mercola, Joseph. http://www.mercola.com.

Morse, Robert, ND. *The Detox Miracle Sourcebook*. Prescott, AZ: Holm Press, 2004.

Myers, Diana. "Colorectal cancer death statistics for the U.S." http://coloncancer.about.com/od/cancerstatistics/a/US _Death_CRC.htm.

National Digestive Diseases Information Clearinghouse. "Constipation." http://www.digestive.niddk.nih.gov/ddiseases/pubs/constipation/index.htm.

———. "Diverticulosis and diverticulitis." http://www.digestive.niddk.nih.gov/ddiseases/pubs/diverticulosis.

Schultz, Richard. *Healing Colon Disease Naturally*. Marina del Rey, CA: Natural Healing Publications, 2003.

Watson, Brenda, ND. *Essential Cleansing for Perfect Health*. Clearwater, FL: Renew Life Press, 2006.

———. *Renew Your Life*. Clearwater, FL: Renew Life Press, 2002.

"What is colorectal cancer?" American Cancer Society. http://www.cancer.org/cancer/colonandrectumcancer/overviewguide/colorectal-cancer-overview-what-is-colorectal-cancer.

## CHAPTER SIX

Anderson, Richard. *The Liver: Cleansing and Rejuvenating the Vital Organ*. Medford, OR: Christobe Publishing, 1999.

Calbom, Cherie, and John Calbom. *The Coconut Diet*. New York: Warner, 2005.

Calbom, Cherie, John Calbom, and Michael Mahaffey. *The Complete Cancer Cleanse*. Nashville, TN: Thomas Nelson, 2003.

National Digestive Diseases Information Clearinghouse. "Gallstones." http://digestive.niddk.nih.gov/ddiseases/pubs/gallstones.

Schulze, Richard. *Healing Liver and Gallbladder Disease Naturally*. Marina del Rey, CA: Natural Healing Publications, 2003.

Watson, Brenda, ND. *Essential Cleansing for Perfect Health*. Clearwater, FL: Renew Life Press, 2006.

## CHAPTER SEVEN

Anderson, Richard. *Cleanse and Purify Thyself.* Book 1.5. Mount Shasta, CA: Triumph Books, 1998.

Bergsson, Gudmundur, Jóhann Arnfinnsson, Ólafur Steingríms-son, and Halldor Thormar. "In vitro killing of *Candida albicans* by fatty acids and monoglycerides." *Antimicrobial Agents and Chemotherapy* 45, no. 11 (November 2001): 3209–12.

Calbom, Cherie, and John Calbom. *The Coconut Diet.* New York: Warner, 2005.

Calbom, Cherie, John Calbom, and Michael Mahaffey. *The Complete Cancer Cleanse.* Nashville, TN: Thomas Nelson, 2003.

Cha, C. W. "A study on the effect of garlic to heavy metal poisoning of rat." *Journal of Korean Medical Science* 2 (1987): 213–23. In *The Encyclopedia of Natural Medicine,* 2nd edition, by Michael Murray and Joseph Pizzorno. Rocklin, CA: Prima Publishing, 1998.

Clarkson, T. W., et al. "The prediction of intake of mercury vapor from amalgam." In *Biological Monitoring of Toxic Metals,* 247–64. New York: Plenum Press, 1988. Also in *Dental Mercury Detox,* revised edition, by Sam Ziff, Michael Ziff, and Mats Hanson. Orlando, FL: Bio-Probe, 1988.

Colbert, Don, MD. *Toxic Relief: Restore Health and Energy Through Fasting and Detoxification.* Lake Mary, FL: Siloam, 2003.

Crook, William G., MD. *The Yeast Connection.* Jackson, TN: Professional Books, 1983, 14.

DiagnoseMe.com. "Parasite infection: overview." http://www.diagnose-me.com/symptoms-of/parasite-infection.html.

Gittleman, Ann Louise. *Natural Healing for Parasites.* New York: Healing Wisdom Publications, 1995.

Kroker, G. F. "Chronic candidiasis and allergy." In *Food Allergy and Intolerance,* edited by J. Brostoff and S. J. Challacombe. Philadelphia: W.B. Saunders, 1987, 850–72.

Mercola, Joseph. "Italian court reignites MMR vaccine debate after award over child with autism." June 25, 2012. http://articles.mercola.com/sites/articles/archive/2012/06/25/mmr-vaccine-caused-autism.aspx.

————. "A victory for health—FDA forced to admit that mercury fillings are hazardous." June 26, 2008. http://articles.mercola.com/sites/articles/archive/2008/06/26/a-victory-for-health-fda-forced-to-admit-that-mercury-fillings-are-hazardous.aspx.

Murray, Michael, ND, and Joseph Pizzorno, ND. *Encyclopedia of Natural Medicine*. Rocklin, CA: Prima Publishing, 1998, 306.

Naiman, Ingrid. "Parasitic infection: symptoms and treatment." KitchenDoctor.com. http://www.kitchendoctor.com/parasite_infection/parasite_symptoms.php.

Truss, O. "The missing diagnosis." In *Encyclopedia of Natural Medicine*, Michael Murray, ND, and Joseph Pizzorno, ND. Rocklin, CA: Prima Publishing, 1998, 300.

Watson, Brenda, ND. *Essential Cleansing for Perfect Health*. Clearwater, FL: Renew Life Press, 2006.

————. *Renew Your Life*. Clearwater, FL: Renew Life Press, 2002.

## CHAPTER EIGHT

Bolt, Martin. *Pursuing Human Strengths*. New York: Worth Publishers, 2004.

Calbom, Cherie, John Calbom, and Michael Mahaffey. *The Complete Cancer Cleanse*. Nashville, TN: Thomas Nelson, 2003.

Cornell, Ann Weiser, PhD. *The Power of Focusing: A Practical Guide to Emotional Self-Healing*. New York: MJF Books, 1996.

Dwoskin, Dale, and Sedona Training Associates. *The Sedona Method Course Workbook: Your Keys to Lasting Happiness, Abundance and Well Being*. Sedona, AR: Sedona Training Associates, 2000.

Hutchison, Michael. *Mega Brain Power: Transform Your Life with Mind Machines and Brain Nutrients*. New York: Hyperion, 1994.

Keyes, Ken, Jr. *Handbook to Higher Consciousness*. 5th edition. St. Mary, KY: Cornucopia Institute, 1975.

Levine, Barbara Hoberman. *Your Body Believes Every Word You Say*. Boulder Creek, CA: Aslan Publishing, 1991.

Matthew 18:21–22. New International Version.

Northrup, Christiane, MD. *Women's Bodies, Women's Wisdom*. New York: Bantam, 1994.

Pert, Candace. *Molecules of Emotion*. New York: Simon & Schuster, 1999.

Sanford, Agnes. *The Healing Light*. New York: Ballantine Books, 1947.

Sanford, John, and Paula Sanford. *The Transformation of the Inner Man*. South Plainfield, NJ: Bridge Publishing, 1982.

Soriano, Rino. "When your emotions become like ticking bombs and cause disease." http://www.ezinearticles.com.

Stokes, Hilary, MSW, MA, and Kim Ward, MA. "The art of forgiveness." *Sanoviv Health Retreat Healing Journal* (1991).

Townsley, Cheryl, ND. *Discovering Wholeness: The Spirit, Soul and Body Connection*. Littleton, CO: LFH Publishing, 2000.

Witvliet, Charlotte van Oyen, T. Ludwig, K. Vander Laan. "Granting forgiveness or harboring grudges: Implications for emotion, physiology, and health." *Psychological Science* 121 (2001): 117–23.

Wright, Henry. *A More Excellent Way*. Thomaston, GA: Pleasant Valley Publications, 1999.

# Acknowledgments

To those who assisted in researching and writing this book, we are forever grateful.

Thank you to Michele Libin, who assisted us in researching and writing this book: we are so very appreciative. You are a dear friend and a valued writer with a wonderful future ahead; thank you for your great contribution to this project.

To our editors Diana Baroni and Leila Porteous, who made this project happen: thank you for your creativity and determination as always to make this book the very best it could be.

To our literary agent Pamela Harty, who once again helped us find a home for our work.

Last, we wish to express our deep and lasting appreciation to all the people, the Holy Trinity, and the angels who have assisted us with this book. To our dear heavenly Father,

Jesus Christ, and Holy Spirit, thank You for guiding us throughout this project. We are so grateful that You showed us Your ways of wisdom and truth as to how to care for the human body. We feel that we've found the fountain of life in the juicing and cleansing programs we've been guided to embrace. Thank You for our health and the awesome responsibility of guiding those who have lost their health, their peace of mind, or their way concerning the care of their bodies. For the healing You've given us and Your unconditional love, we are so very grateful.

# Index

# About the Authors

**CHERIE CALBOM, MS, CN,** is known as a leading expert on nutrition. She earned a master of science degree in nutrition from Bastyr University. She frequently appears on television and speaks nationwide on the benefits of juicing and healthy living. She is author of twenty-one books, including the best sellers *The Juice Lady's Big Book of Juices and Green Smoothies*, *The Juice Turbo Diet*, *The Juice Lady's Living Foods Revolution*, *The Juice Lady's Guide to Juicing for Health*, *The Coconut Diet*, and *The Ultimate Smoothie Book*. Cherie and her husband, John, conduct Health and Wellness Juice Retreats in Santa Fe, New Mexico, where they live.

**JOHN CALBOM, MA,** is director of Trinity Retreat house, president of Trinity Wellness Institute, and a certified Heart-Math provider. He is a behavioral medicine specialist, psychotherapist, and Eastern Orthodox priest. He was vice president of St. Luke Medical Center and worked as a behavioral medicine therapist in complementary and preventive medicine.